ON C

LABORATORY MEDICINE
and PATHOLOGY

Other titles in the On Call series

ON CALL

LABORATORY MEDICINE and PATHOLOGY

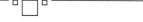

JOHN BERNARD HENRY, MD
Distinguished Service Professor
Director, Pathology 200
College of Medicine

Director, Transfusion Medicine and Transfusion Medicine Fellowship
Hemapheresis, HLA, Progenitor Cell and Parentage Testing
Laboratories

Attending Pathologist
University Hospital
State University of New York
Upstate Medical University
Syracuse, New York

□ □ □

SHARAD C. MATHUR, MD
Instructor in Pathology
College of Medicine
Fellow in Hematopathology
University Hospital
State University of New York
Upstate Medical University
Syracuse, New York

W.B. SAUNDERS COMPANY
A Division of Harcourt Brace & Company
Philadelphia London New York Toronto St. Louis Sydney

W.B. SAUNDERS COMPANY
A Division of Harcourt Brace & Company

The Curtis Center
Independence Square West
Philadelphia, Pennsylvania 19106

Library of Congress Cataloging-in-Publication Data

Henry, John Bernard, 1928-
On call laboratory medicine and pathology / John Bernard Henry, Sharad C. Mathur.

p.; cm.—(On call series)

Includes bibliographical references and index.

ISBN 0-7216-9004-1 (alk. paper)

1. Diagnosis, Laboratory—Handbooks, manuals, etc. I. Title: Laboratory
   medicine and pathology. II. Mathur, Sharad C. III. Title. IV. Series.
   [DNLM: a. Laboratory Techniques and Procedures—Handbooks.
   2. Emergencies—Handbooks. QY 39 H522o 2000]

RB38.2 .H46 2000

616.07956—dc21   00-023911

Cover illustration is a detail from the painting *Takeoff*, glass enamel on steel, by Virgil Cantini, PhD, with permission from the artist.

ON CALL LABORATORY
MEDICINE AND PATHOLOGY   ISBN 0-7216-9004-1

Printed in the United States of America

Last digit is the print number: 9 8 7 6 5 4 3 2 1

To our wives
Georgette and Sangeeta

□ □ □

FOREWORD

For more than 92 years the textbook entitled *Clinical Diagnosis and Management by Laboratory Methods* has been the major reference for residents in pathology, medical technology students, and clinicians. The purpose of that textbook was to provide a comprehensive review of the entire field of clinical pathology and laboratory medicine. However, for a long time there has been a significant need for a pocket-sized manual to assist the pathology resident on call in fulfilling his or her responsibilities in a timely fashion. Most other disciplines of medicine have enjoyed such a book for one or two generations. Fortunately Dr. John Bernard Henry, the current editor of the *Clinical Diagnosis and Management by Laboratory Methods*, and Dr. Sharad Mathur, the fellow in hematopathology and former pathology resident at the SUNY Health Science Center, have joined together to fill the gap and present a thorough but succinctly written pocket-sized book to assist the pathology resident on call in both anatomic pathology and clinical pathology.

This book is based on the evolving responsibilities of the pathology resident on call at our institution for more than 35 years. The focus of the book is on the consultative activities of the pathology residents with residents and attendings in other medical and surgical disciplines. This book should facilitate prompt and appropriate support to our clinical colleagues through whom we serve most of our patients. It should help anyone obtain the most out of the laboratory in an efficient manner when assistance is needed most rapidly during evenings, nights, weekends, and holidays. The resident and attending pathologist on call can receive, through this manual, information that will help them become confident and competent particularly when practicing outside one's special expertise. It should also facilitate learning and more responsive patient care service. This book captures the essence of "what a pathologist does" in an abbreviated manner to allow more access to the clinical laboratories in a timely manner. Most importantly it responds to the need for structured learning during the on-call hours. It should become a benchmark text and resource in the graduate medical education of pathologists.

Frederick R. Davey, MD
Professor and Chairman
Department of Pathology
SUNY Upstate Medical University
Syracuse, New York

PREFACE

An integral, important, substantive part of learning for pathology residents and one that concurrently provides critical, timely patient care service occurs when residents are on call. Indeed, this is the time, especially nights, weekends, and holidays, that offers a major portion of unique challenging clinical problems for prompt resolution in a concise, comprehensive, and efficient manner through laboratory medicine and pathology. The in-depth, sequential resident rotations in anatomic and clinical pathology especially in sections of Blood Bank and Transfusion Medicine, Hematology and Coagulation, Chemistry, Microscopy, Microbiology, Immunology, Cytogenetics, Molecular Pathology, Surgical Pathology, Forensic and Autopsy Pathology, Neuropathology, and Cytopathology are the foundation of an integrated and holistic clinical laboratory response to patient problems and clinician needs that occur when the residents are on call and in the day-to-day practice of pathologists, often in an urgent or emergent-response environment.

This pocket-sized abbreviated text, *On Call Laboratory Medicine and Pathology*, laden with tables and figures, reflects brevity in a comprehensive approach to clinical pathology medical problem solving and patient assessment for hospitalized and ambulatory patients most frequently encountered when residents and attending pathologists are on call. It should provide a measure of confidence to such residents and attending pathologists. It reflects our approach, which has evolved over 30 years and is compiled annually in our *Residency Program Description Manual* and *Pathology Manual*. It is the "call" responsibilities and duties described in these manuals that provide a point of departure for this compendium.

On Call Laboratory Medicine and Pathology incorporates a dual approach—both from a section or division of laboratory service from which laboratory information and data emerge as well as from specific clinical challenges of patient care requiring diagnostic and management support in medical problem solving. These often unique and complex medical problem-solving demands prevail within and among laboratory sections; although some are virtually exclusive to one section, others draw upon several sections for the resolution of a single patient medical problem. Hence, one can use *On Call Laboratory Medicine and Pathology* starting either from a patient medical problem (most often articulated by a resident or attending physician) or from a call from a technologist in the laboratory. However, nurse practitioners, physician assistants, medical students, and physicians other than pathologists should also find

On Call Laboratory Medicine and Pathology useful for their specific medical problem solving in both diagnosis and management.

The clinical laboratory is the major contributor of hard scientific information (growing exponentially) to a patient's medical record and care that occurs 24 hours a day and 7 days a week. Through residents and pathologists on call, this *On Call Laboratory Medicine and Pathology* pocketbook text literally provides round-the-clock support to patients through their clinicians. It concurrently should assist pathology residents learning during graduate medical education as well as practicing pathologists and others who desire a quick resource for review in the care of their patients. Finally, it will also provide both confidence and a resource for decision making and responding.

Providing accessible, organized responses to the assessment and management of clinical problems wherever they arise through laboratory medicine is central to this text. A guide to responding to calls and queries when one is on call coupled with a succinct focus of a core of information as a response to clinical problem solving through laboratory medicine is the major goal of this handbook. It is more on how to get the most out of the laboratory than on principles and practice of laboratory medicine. However, it will serve pathologists and virtually any practitioner who cares for patients in diagnosis and management as a quick reference though not a definitive resource of clinical pathology.

We are indebted to our residents and many colleagues and friends who have generously shared their thoughts and approaches to core information and clinical problem solving through *On Call Laboratory Medicine And Pathology.*

We accept full responsibility for any errors of omission or commission and welcome any comments, reactions, or suggestions to make the next edition more useful to readers.

John Bernard Henry
Sharad C. Mathur

ACKNOWLEDGMENTS

To all resident and attending physicians in Clinical Pathology who functioned as a team of two for 1 week at a time while at the State University of New York, University Hospital for over 35 years and performed on-call responsibilities in a progressive and expanding manner, we are eternally grateful. We express our gratitude for their efforts that have made being on call in Laboratory Medicine and Pathology a patient care service, a learning-teaching experience, and a source of stimulation to all faculty and residents participating in weekly review sessions for "on call" of a prior week.

Dr. Frederick Davey's sustained support for this endeavor and thorough review of the entire manuscript with helpful comments brought this work to its completion. Several individuals were most helpful in providing critical review and comments. Gregory Tetrault, MD, was most helpful in reviewing and commenting on quality assurance. Ann Marie Kazee, MD, provided a helpful critique and review of hemapheresis, and Ms. Karla Lauenstein, MS, MT, (ASCP), SBB, DLM, performed with meticulous attention to detail a review that was most helpful in Transfusion Medicine. Ms. Charlene Hubbell's assistance and report generation in HLA/solid organ transplantation with sustained support were most important.

Ultimately it was Ms. Kay Mevec's enthusiastic response in generating the drafts and final manuscript for our work that brought it to its culmination. Ms. Joan Hough and Ms. Judy Kelsey provided critical support that expedited this endeavor and made it possible for it to happen in a timely manner.

Undoubtedly there are others who have contributed, particularly our attending physicians and several generations of technical and clerical staff in generating the two manuals that we have borrowed from heavily in this endeavor, i.e., the July 1998–1999 and 1999–2000 *Pathology Manual* and the *Residency Program Description Manual.* We are indebted to them and our several colleagues as contributors to the nineteenth edition of *Clinical Diagnosis and Management by Laboratory Methods.*

To Carl Masthay for his sustained, meticulous, excellent editorial effort with a keen sense of humor and to William R. Schmitt for his overarching superior editorial guidance and direction as Editorial Manager, W.B. Saunders Company, we are most grateful.

John Bernard Henry, MD
Sharad Mathur, MD

CONTENTS

COMMON CALLS IN ANATOMIC PATHOLOGY

APPENDIX A REFERENCE INTERVALS (NORMAL VALUES) AND SI UNITS

APPENDIX B COMMON FIXATIVES IN SURGICAL PATHOLOGY

APPENDIX C COMMON EPONYMOUS TESTS AND DETERMINATIONS

ON CALL

LABORATORY MEDICINE
and PATHOLOGY

HOW TO GET THE MOST
OUT OF THE CLINICAL
LABORATORY

APPROACH TO ON-CALL PROBLEMS

CLINICAL PATHOLOGY
ANATOMIC PATHOLOGY

■ CLINICAL PATHOLOGY

To respond promptly, effectively and efficiently to a "call" from a clinical colleague, it is important to understand the needs and expectations sought. These range from diagnosis, management, and specific therapy to identifying etiology, complication, or sequela of disease (Fig. 1–1). The request may be for best-available measurement or examination to confirm a clinical impression or rule out a disease, or to how quickly a specific determination or blood component for therapy can be made available. It may be an attention call for a consultation in anticipation of a new admission that may require therapeutic hemapheresis. Finally, the "call" may be for help in what to do with a specimen (collect and transport) or what to do next to solve a problem, that is, what test or tests and in what order and how long it will require.

Asking the right question in response to the call for clarification or confirmation is central to a quick turnaround time (TAT), often so important in patient care. Recall or reference to Fig. 1–1 may help you pinpoint a particular aspect of illness at issue and anticipate other subsequent needs promptly.

Your response will be measured in terms of quality (accuracy, specificity, and completeness) and turnaround time (TAT), hence the importance of understanding the "call" thoroughly at the beginning. Equally important is your knowledge and full appreciation of the laboratory resources available (people, technology and instrumentation, blood products and derivatives, test menu with specimen requirements) coupled with current status of quality assurance (QA), especially quality control (QC), and overall operations (demands with quick response) at the time.

Morning and afternoon rounds on weekdays as well as on weekend or holiday mornings in the laboratory through MBWA (management by walking around) and listening and talking to staff and associates will provide such insight and awareness of both operations and resources with identification of actual or potential problems. It is also the time to seek out abnormal peripheral blood smears, positive blood or catheter and line cultures, cerebrospinal or other body fluids with abnormal findings or positive cultures, crystals in joint fluids, and abnormal urinary sediments. Follow-up on such patients with or through attending and resident physicians should be accomplished, including a patient visit with a medical record review if necessary for further clarification.

When you may not have all the answers or be confident, it is all right to say, "I don't know, but I will get back to you right away," or specify the time you estimate. Therefore, pathology residents on call require an attending pathologist on call as a backup and educational support. Consultation with your attending physician or speaking with a technical staff member may be all that is required at the time. Of course, the attending pathologist should meet with you and review at first hand any examination or measurement that requires confirmation. This may also include seeing the patient and speaking with a clinician or clinicians to ascertain further the patient's needs and provide a better match with laboratory resources available. Of course, further consultation with an "expert" or sub-

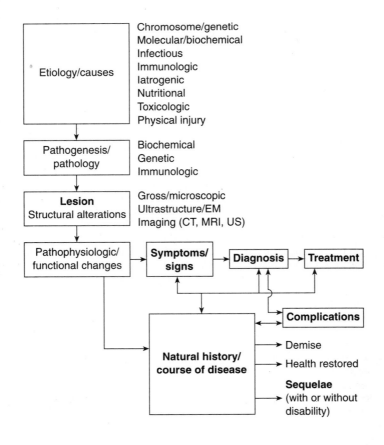

specialist in the department may also be in order. General pathologists on call in their hospital have the same access to their pathology colleagues as experts as well.

However, there is no substitute for an in-depth knowledge of the patient's disease (see Fig. 1–1) and needs derived firsthand from

---

Figure 1–1 □ Unifying concept of disease for on call. "Call" begins with the arrival of a new patient, a "41-year-old mother with a leukocyte count of 340,000/μL, anemia, and a severe headache"; anticipate the need to establish the diagnosis of leukemia with a complete blood count (CBC) and bone marrow examinations. Patient was admitted to Hematology-Oncology Service with her initial contact made to pathology's resident on call. The attending pathologist on call will also review bone marrow examination and peripheral blood examination with resident to confirm diagnosis of acute myelogenous leukemia (AML) moving from *lesion* to *diagnosis* (as in this figure). *Treatment* is invoked with a leukocyte count of 340,000/μL necessitating hemapheresis as leukapheresis for cytoreduction followed by chemotherapy over several weeks. This figure also accommodates *symptoms and signs* (headache and leukemoid reaction) with the *diagnosis* of AML, anemia, and thrombocytopenia. *Treatment* requirements ensue and include arranging for a vascular access catheter (because of observed marginal peripheral venous access) to be inserted by available interventional radiologist or surgeon in view of diagnosis of AML, anticipating several weeks of chemotherapy and a potential candidate for autogeneic or allogeneic peripheral blood progenitor cell transplantation. Catheter should be ordered accordingly as a permanent rather than a temporary catheter. Next, the apheresis nurse is called in after obtainment of a completed consultation form for the aphersis procedure followed by an informed consent with the patient. *Complications* in the figure include leukostasis and possible DIC with bleeding, thrombosis, and anemia along with the likelihood of hypocalcemia (citrate induced). During leukapheresis treatment, a goal of 60% reduction of WBC with or without reduction in WBC (decrease to 100,000/μL) is established. After a patient history and a physical examination are performed, findings are recorded in the patient's medical record, incorporating assessment, diagnosis, and management plan with appropriate written orders. Since leukapheresis is a medical emergency requiring one or two successive procedures over 2 days, contemplate further to avoid other *complications* and *sequelae.* Review of this figure should also prompt initiation of cytogenetic studies to clarify or refine the *diagnosis, lesion,* and *cause. Pathogenesis* was noteworthy in its brevity "less than 1 week of URI and 2 days of headache and weakness/fatigue" of *symptoms* and *signs* of anemia. Throughout, there is close collaboration with clinical colleagues (hematology-oncology, radiology, surgery, and nursing), with oral and written communication of your needs and also responding to patient's needs. By this time, two hemapheresis nurses have arrived to initiate first procedure with appropriate direction and support. A postprocedure medical-record progress note should include outcome (WBC reduction attained as number and percentage), catheter flow rate changes or hypocalcemia problems encountered, and how they were managed. The note is concluded with patient assessment and plan, including time of next procedure if anticipated with next-day preprocedure orders in medical chart.

seeing the patient, as well as through others, to provide the most effective laboratory response and support.

■ ANATOMIC PATHOLOGY

On-call responsibilities are a valuable part of the learning experience that residency training and an attending pathologist provide. The ability to handle "calls" in a prompt and effective manner is crucial to establish one's status as a "consultant," which is essentially the role of pathologists in such situations.

In Anatomic Pathology, "call" involves intraoperative consultation, cytology, autopsy, and miscellaneous tissue handling or processing issues. Although it is not our intent to discuss the techniques employed in these calls (topics that are discussed at length in excellent references), a few points deserve mention regarding the overall approach to Anatomic Pathology calls.

Understanding the needs and expectations of our clinical colleagues is, as with a Clinical Pathology "call," the essence in providing the best service possible. Although turnaround time (TAT) may be of prime importance in an intraoperative consultation with the patient under anesthesia, a laborious and time-consuming dissection of the heart (after adequate fixation) may be the most important part of a weekend autopsy of a child with congenital heart disease. Thus it is imperative to clearly and comprehensively establish what exactly the clinical question that needs to be answered or goal to be pursued is before one formulates the mode of action. As discussed in subsequent chapters, the handling of autopsy cases and intraoperative consultations will vary widely depending on the information sought and may involve different tissue processing and fixation requirements to fit the examination or analytic needs anticipated at a later date.

Technical skills cannot be learned through reading alone, and therefore each resident must master the art of frozen sections, fine-needle aspirations (FNA), autopsy dissections, and other such procedures by performing as many as possible under the guidance of more senior pathologists. It is certainly desirable to acquire basic skills in these areas and to familiarize oneself with departmental protocols before taking a call. Within the current environment of regulations, accreditation, and licensing, an attending pathologist's review is essential in most diagnostic decisions, and therefore call situations are also excellent opportunities to interact with and learn from your attendings in pathology as well as from clinical colleagues.

In summary, being on call is providing patient care service, serving as a consultant, managing the laboratory, and learning through a progressive assumption of responsibility so important in graduate and continuing medical education. You must respond to patient problems and clinician needs "call" in a manner that reflects the science of disease and practice of laboratory medicine and pathology.

2

COMMUNICATING WITH COLLEAGUES

Communicating **verbally** (that is, either *orally* or *in writing*), as well as by body language, is crucial to getting the most out of the laboratory. In every verbal communication, there are four conversations: (1) what you said, (2) what you assume you said, (3) what the other person heard, and (4) what the other person believes he or she heard. In other words, never be surprised when an error in communication arises and try to minimize if not eliminate such errors through meticulous attention to selection of words, pertinent questions, and repetition and by summarizing conclusions for the other person for validation.

Your attitude must reflect your understanding of "call" as a commitment to respond in the most expeditious manner to meet the needs of patients. As laboratorians, we are here to serve and support our clinical colleagues. We can do that best when we appreciate fully their needs and expectations. "Get the message right the first time" is an old axiom that is so true in communication in medicine.

We serve most of our patients through and with other physicians as our clinical colleagues. However, our customers include patients, physicians, nurses, nurse practitioners (NP), and physician assistants (PA). Communication with each and with our technical, clerical, and administrative staff are all important in terms of content clarity and precision and must be conducted in a respectful manner.

Consultation and laboratory request forms are examples of **written** communications that must be developed with great care and attention to detail to assure that essential information is available to respond to a request for service. Both clinician and patient will benefit more in terms of quality, completeness, and promptness of response and support when such forms are completed fully and legibly. In our therapeutic hemapheresis consultation form, pertinent clinical information—including diagnoses, medications, and anticipated need for removal of a specific constituent with patient's hematocrit, leukocyte, and platelet counts along with weight (kg) and height (cm)—are requisite to our response. Likewise, laboratory request forms should facilitate the clinician's identification of specific measurements and examinations relevant to the patient's medical problem or problems, including organ and disease panels of selected determinations with appropriate specificity and sensitivity coupled with cost effectiveness to generate results most efficiently. This is more challenging today in view of regulations and reimbursement requiring medical necessity and International Classification of Diseases (ICD-9) diagnosis codes.

Informed consent from the patient for procedures and blood-product infusion should likewise be accomplished with great care; appropriate forms including risks and benefits incorporating signatures of patient, attending physician, and witness are important documents, especially when annotated appropriately with any patient reservations or specific concerns.

Face-to-face and telephone interactions, coupled with electronic mail (e-mail) and written correspondence including follow-up to consultations, deserve special attention according to circumstances. In turn, each form of communication is a unique opportunity to reflect favorably upon yourself, your service, the department of pathology and laboratory medicine, as well as the institution or organization.

Patient needs should always come first in our response to support our clinical colleagues. If in doubt or if an extended debate ensues over a single measurement or examination, "do it" and resolve the issue the next day or following Monday morning.

Always keep in mind that a clinician or anyone else who calls to your attention what he or she perceives as an error in a report or result is doing you and the laboratory a real favor. Colleagues can and do differ from one another in their opinion or interpretation; it is more than acceptable to receive, hear, and understand what may be a difference in opinion or interpretation. This is most vivid in a consultation interchange or interaction. Thank that person for their call and proceed to resolve it without accepting or denying fault. (See Chapter 4.)

A Monday morning patient care service rounds or conference is an excellent opportunity for a resident on call (with attending on call present) for the prior week and for all pathology residents and attending staff to have a review, discussion, and comment for each "call" received sequentially and serially for the on-call time or week (Fig. 2–1). Pertinent clinical and laboratory information or data for each patient "call" is presented or projected by the resident on call along with the nature of the "call" and response. Experts can then comment or be quizzed on the spot to confirm or modify the action or response taken with follow-up notes in the patient record if appropriate. A clerical staff record of each call is summarized for the record as minutes for what is almost uniformly an excellent teaching and learning experience for all present. This also serves as a record of patient care that benefits specific patients then and all patients subsequently (see Fig. 2–1).

Communication is a manifestation of good leadership and management. Managers make appropriate or right decisions in a timely manner through planning, organizing, staffing, directing, and controlling (following through on direction). Although leaders

CLINICAL PATHOLOGY-SERVICE REVIEW
Monday, 11 AM, UH 3816

ADMINISTRATIVE REPORT:

1. Instrument or test failures. (What was the nature of the failure? What was done to correct it? Were there any adverse patient consequences?)

2. Personnel problems. (Absenteeism? Inability to handle work load in a specific section?)

3. Miscellaneous administrative problems. (Turnaround-time problems, call-ins, and problems with quality assurance.)

ANNOUNCEMENTS:

FOLLOW-UP OF CALLS/PROBLEMS FROM PREVIOUS WEEKS:*

NEW CALLS/PROBLEMS THIS PAST WEEK:*

INTERESTING CASE(S):*

_____   _____/_____
Date   Resident/Attending

*Attach brief synopsis of case(s)

Figure 2–1 □ Clinical Pathology service review.

identify the direction (goals), managers provide the support (objectives) to get things done through and with other people. In the end, it is how many things you get done as well as how quickly that counts. In laboratory medicine and pathology, residents and attending physicians on call can make it all happen to serve even better our patients and clinical colleagues. Eventually the "Virtual Clinical Laboratory" with a patient's pertinent clinical information with laboratory results and reports on the World Wide Web site (www) will exist for all pathologists and their clinical colleagues. This will facilitate communication for both clinicians and pathologists over a patient's laboratory results and expedite medical problem solving together on line during real time through pathologist and clinician interaction. Translation, interpretation, and most appropriate selection and sequence of optimal laboratory testing (measurements and examinations) for a particular patient's medical problem can be available to expedite patient care. A pathologist can serve even better his or her clinical colleague when he or she has available relevant clinical information and can observe the configuration (variety) of tests selected and the trends in laboratory data. Clinicians can secure more promptly a confirmation of the test selection for optimal sensitivity, specificity in disease detection, diagnosis, and management. This will be the ultimate in communication and collaboration and is already evolving to the benefit of patients and our clinical colleagues.

3

LABORATORY MEASUREMENTS AND EXAMINATIONS:
Strengths and Limitations

SENSITIVITY AND SPECIFICITY

There is no such thing as a simple test. Indeed, each determination is fraught with potential pitfalls, including test-order entry; patient preparation (fasting or special diet, timing, posture, medications); patient identification; specimen collection, labeling, transport, storage, and processing; result reporting; and interpretation of laboratory reports. A problem with any of those steps may produce clinically significant errors that have nothing to do with accuracy and precision of testing. Testing (analytic) errors are rare because of automation and standardization of methods, the quality of work from competent and well-trained laboratorians following standard operating procedures (SOPs) and implementation of appropriate quality control (QC) and quality assurance (QA) protocols that include external proficiency testing (PT). The testing process and therefore laboratory QA begin with the clinician ordering a test on a patient and end with the clinician treating the patient based, in part, on test results. These factors must be considered by the pathologist when receiving a "call" that questions laboratory results that do not appear to correlate with the patient's condition. The response to such a "call" must include meticulous attention to details and steps in the entire process or system, and if there remains any doubt, a "confirmation request" should ensue (Chapter 4). Specimen retention (sera, plasma) and proper storage for 7 days and whole blood for 24 hours facilitate a repeat measurement and validation.

However, it is safe to assume with reasonable confidence and medical certainty that a measurement or examination is valid until proved otherwise in view of today's laboratory medicine and pathology science and technology with dedicated, competent staff embracing QA and SOPs. Not only is there an internal ongoing review daily of methodology and analytical systems by pathologists, associates or assistants, and technical staff (also examining QA, QC, and PT) but also a focused intensive study of individual patients periodically that can make manifest any pitfalls or random errors. This sharpens the clinical relevance of laboratory medicine and pathology in the reality of day-to-day patient care. Certification and demonstration of continuing competency of personnel at all levels is integral and ongoing. External laboratory reviews for accreditation associated with detailed inspection including PT are regular occurrences, often in the form of unannounced visits to further assure public and payers that a high-quality laboratory service is in place.

Unfortunately, most problems, reported errors, or questionable results are attributable to nonanalytical causes, with the potential for analytical errors being greater today than in the past because of marginal staffing as a cost-cutting effort.

Just as there is no such thing as a simple test, there is no such thing as a perfect test or determination. Each assay, though accurate and precise, with a coefficient of variation (CV) of about 5% (CV = 5%), reflects each measurement as a compromise in terms of sensitivity and specificity (see below). Most routine tests have CVs less than 5% for results in the normal range, some tests have higher CVs for low results (e.g., PSA, TSH, and folate), and a few tests always have larger CVs (e.g., estradiol, cortisol, and some enzymes). A few measurements have CVs in the 1–2% range (some automated chemistry assays and automated blood cell counts).

Precision reflects analytical variation about the mean of a measurement, i.e., reproducibility of the method. Such precision is determined and available for each measurement as a CV, expressed as

$$\left(\frac{SD}{Mean} \right)$$

The precision of most measurements is usually less than plus or minus five percent coefficient of variation (CV = ±5%), and, as stated, relatively few measurements exceed a CV of 5%, and so it is a dependable guide in the evaluation of a single test result. Since the numerical value of the CV for each test result is about ±5% of the result value, if exceeded, it represents a significant change in the patient versus a change in the laboratory in day-to-day or longer intervals. About two thirds of the laboratory data are applied in patient management rather than in diagnosis. Precision or reproducibility is thus more important than accuracy though accuracy is still of the utmost importance and challenge, especially for constituents in minimal concentration, e.g., hormones. Hence for most constituents there is a great emphasis in clinical pathology data review to consider day-to-day variation in a result value within or exceeding a CV of 5% for detection of a real change in a patient requiring management attention. One does not have to memorize mean and standard deviation (SD), e.g., mean ± 2 SDs for a 95% confidence interval, to ascertain the change in a single patient value; applying a CV = 5% plus or minus value is sufficient if you keep in mind the exceptions noted. In the laboratory, delta (or 'change') check values are established by the director based on a combination of method precision, within patient biologic variation and clinical needs. Daily checks for patient values that lie significantly outside of their established reference intervals or have undergone large changes over a 24-hour period are reported as "failed delta checks." Thus patients with significant abnormal laboratory findings can be identified. Laboratory staff and pathologists use delta checks, and clinically significant differences are used by pathologists and clinicians. In addition, computer application programs that can evaluate clinical and laboratory findings to generate differential diagnoses are now available.

■ SENSITIVITY AND SPECIFICITY

The sensitivity of a test is the probability that a person with a particular disease will have an abnormal result. Specificity in turn means that a person without a particular disease will have a normal result or value. In other words, virtually no determination is 100% sensitive for detection and 100% specific for a single disease or pathologic process.

Both sensitivity and specificity are, however, affected by the prevalence of a particular disease. When sensitivity and specificity are used with prevalence of a particular disease, the predictive value of a measurement or examination can be ascertained. Without knowledge of the prevalence of a disease in a particular patient, the power of a predictive value is not readily available. Since the prevalence of many diseases is unavailable, test selection is based on clinical judgment with a best estimate of prevalence and an awareness of test specificity and sensitivity. Matching clinical assessment with selection of laboratory determinations is a challenge at times. Several tests may complement and supplement one another because there can be an overlap with validation of a single most-important determination. Therefore a panel or profile of selected measurements and examinations that fit a particular clinical problem, pathologic process, or disease can save time (TAT) on the way to clinical diagnosis or treatment and, with proper selection of technology or instrumentation, be cost effective. Appropriate charges should recognize the total cost of tests selected for organ panels or disease profiles (Table 3–1), which lend themselves to interpretation, analysis, and test validation. This can be the most cost-effective and efficient use of the laboratory in medical care, health assessment, and wellness promotion.

Organ panels and disease profiles also fit with optimal laboratory utilization. Who can better match technology and other laboratory resources available for patient diseases and organ or system specificity than pathologists, especially when on call? It is often as important to know what measurements and examinations are negative (normal) or within reference intervals (normal values) as those tests that are positive (abnormal) in the care of a single

Text continued on page 18

Table 3–1 □ CLINICAL PATHOLOGY PANELS

Anemia

CBC with indices, reticulocyte count and microscopic examination
Microcytic: *Iron panel,* ESR
Normocytic: ESR, *hemolysis profile*
Macrocytic: B_{12}, folate, TSH

Arterial Blood Gas

pH	P_aO_2
P_aCO_2	CO_2 content
O_2 saturation	$P_{A-a}O_2$

Arthritis

ESR (sedimentation rate)	C-reactive protein
Uric acid	Rheumatoid factor
ANA	

Bone/Joint

Albumin	Protein, total
Calcium	Uric acid
Phosphorus	Alkaline phosphatase
Osteocalcin	

Cardiac Injury*

Creatine kinase (CK)	Myoglobin
CK-MB	Troponin-I

Chem. Path. 7

Sodium	Potassium
Chloride	Bicarbonate
BUN	Creatinine
Glucose	

Coagulation Screening

Prothrombin time	Platelet count
Thrombin time	Bleeding time
Partial thromboplastin time	

Collagen Disease/SLE

ESR	ANA
C-reactive protein	Anti-DNA
C_3	C_4
ANCA (antineutrophil cytoplasmic antibody)	

Coma

Chem. Path. 7	*Arterial blood gas profile*
Toxicology screen	Alcohol
Salicylate	Lactic acid
Ammonia	Calcium (total and ionized)
Anion gap	Serum osmolality

DIC

Platelet count	Prothrombin time
Thrombin time	Partial thromboplastin time

*Troponin-I (cTn I) will eventually replace CK-MB in Cardiac Injury panel. CK-MB determination on initial patient serum may clarify same initial specimen elevation of cTn I and classify appropriately a patient with a myocardial injury in the previous week.

Table 3–1 □ **CLINICAL PATHOLOGY PANELS** *Continued*

DIC *Continued*

Fibrinogen
Fibrin split products

CBC with examination of blood
   film

Diabetes Mellitus Management

Chem. Path. 7
Hemoglobin A$_{1c}$

Anion gap
Lipid profile

Electrolyte/Fluid Management

Chem. Path. 7
Plasma and urine osmolality
Creatinine clearance
Free water clearance

Anion gap

Enteral/Parenteral Nutrition Management

Chem. Path. 7
Magnesium
Albumin and total protein
Alkaline phosphatase

Calcium
Phosphorus
Triglyceride
Prealbumin
CBC

General Health

CBC
Lipid profile
Albumin
LD
Calcium
Bilirubin, total

Chem. Path. 7
Uric acid
Total protein
AST (GOT)
Alkaline phosphatase
GGT

Hemolysis

CBC
Bilirubin
Haptoglobin
Free hemoglobin (serum and
   urine)

LD
Antiglobulin (direct and
   indirect)
Reticulocyte count

Hepatitis Serology, Acute

Hepatitis A IgM Ab
Hepatitis C Ab

Hepatitis B surface Ag
Hepatitis B core IgM Ab

Hepatitis Serology, Chronic Carrier

Hepatitis Be Ab
Hepatitis B surface Ag

Hepatitis Be Ag
Hepatitis C Ab

HIV

HIV Ab (ELISA) with Western blot confirmation
CBC with CD4 and CD8 lymphocyte subsets

Hypertension

Chem. Path. 7
Urinary free cortisol
Renin

Thyroid screening panel
Urinary metanephrines
Urinalysis

Table continued on following page

Table 3–1 □ CLINICAL PATHOLOGY PANELS *Continued*

Iron

Serum iron
TIBC (total iron-binding)
  capacity)

% Saturation
Ferritin

Lipid, Fasting

Triglycerides
HDL-cholesterol

Total cholesterol
LDL-cholesterol

Liver Function

Albumin
Prothrombin time
Bilirubin (total and direct)
GGT

Protein, total
AST (GOT)
ALT (GPT)
Alkaline phosphatase

Newborn Screening (NY State)

Phenylalanine (phenylketonuria)
Leucine (branched-chain ketonuria)
Galactose-1-phosphate uridyl transferase (galactosemia)
Methionine (homocystinuria)
Thyroxine, TSH (hypothyroidism)
Hemoglobin electrophoresis (sickle cell)
Biotinidase (biotinidase deficiency)

Pancreatic

Amylase
Calcium (total and ionized)
Triglycerides

Lipase
Glucose

Parathyroid

Albumin
Alkaline phosphatase
Magnesium
Creatinine
PTH (whole molecule, amino terminal)

Protein, total
Calcium (total and ionized)
Phosphorus
Urinary calcium

Prenatal Screening

CBC
BUN
Uric acid
ABO and Rh typing
Urinalysis
Toxoplasmosis Ab
CMV Ab
Hepatitis B surface Ag
Cervical Pap smear
Cervical cultures for GC, *Chlamydia,* group B streptococci

Glucose
Creatinine
Free T_4
Antibody screen
Urine culture
Rubella titer
VDRL
Herpes simplex I & II Ab

Renal

Chem. Path. 7
Magnesium
Albumin
24-hr urine protein
Creatinine clearance

Calcium (total and ionized)
Phosphorus
Protein, total
24-hr urine creatinine
CBC

Thyroid Screening

Thyroxine (free T_4)

TSH (third or fourth generation)

Table 3–1 □ CLINICAL PATHOLOGY PANELS *Continued*

Clinical Pathology Panels

Toxicology Screening (urine)

Amphetamines	Barbiturates
Benzodiazepines	Cocaine metabolites
Marijuana metabolites	Methadone
Methaqualone	Opiate metabolites
Phencyclidine	Propoxyphene

Transplant

HIV Ab	HTLV-1 Ab
CMV Ab	VDRL
HSV I and II Ab	EBV capsid Ag and IgG Ab
ABO and Rh typing	Antibody screen
Hepatitis B surface Ag	Hepatitis C Ab
Rubella immune status	
Hepatitis A Ab total and IgM	
HLA typing: A, B, DR, and crossmatch	
Lymphocytotoxic antibody screen	

From Henry JB: Clinical Diagnosis and Management by Laboratory Methods, 19th ed. Philadelphia, WB Saunders Co, 1996.

Final selection for ambulatory and inpatient use of the most cost-effective, sensitive, and specific measurements for each panel should be based on available laboratory technology and appropriate medical staff consultation with the Director of Laboratories in the context of relevant Practice Parameters* and Practice Guidelines. Use for hospitalized patients may be incorporated into "critical pathways" that are evolving.

*Development of Practice Parameters: Principles of Practice Parameters. Chicago, American Medical Association, 1995, pp 1–18. (See order number below.)

Glenn GC: Practice Parameter on Laboratory Panel Testing for Screening and Case Findings in Asymptomatic Adults, Arch Pathol Lab Med 1996;120(10); 929–943.

Henry JB: Focused profiling: Selection of laboratory measurements and examinations. Videotape or 35-mm slides. Wilmington, E.I. du Pont de Nemours & Co., 1982.

Henry JB, Arras MJ: Organ panels: An innovation in health care delivery. Med Times 1970; 98:106.

Henry JB, Howanitz PJ: Organ panels and the relationship of the laboratory to the physician. *In* Young DS, Uddin D, Nipper H, et al (eds), King JS (exec ed): Clinician and Chemist: Proceedings of the First Arnold O. Beckman Conference in Clinical Chemistry. Washington, DC, American Association for Clinical Chemistry, 1979.

Henry JB, Howanitz PJ: Organ panels and the relationship of the laboratory to the physician. *In* AMA Council on Scientific Affairs: Laboratory Tests in Medical Practice, Chicago, 1980.

*Order number OP271693
American Medical Association
P.O. Box 7046
Dover, DE 19903

Table 3–2 □ ORGAN/DISEASE PANELS COMPOSITION AND CURRENT PROCEDURAL TERMINOLOGY CODES (YEAR 2000)

1. Basic metabolic panel—80048

    Glucose—82947
    Calcium—82310
    Creatinine—82565
    Urea nitrogen (BUN)—84520
    Sodium—84295
    Potassium—84132
    Carbon Dioxide—82374
    Chloride—82435

2. Comprehensive metabolic panel —80053

    AST, SGOT—84450
    ALT, SGPT—84460
    Bilirubin, total—82247
    Phosphatase, alkaline—84075
    Protein, total—84155
    Albumin—82040
    Glucose—82947
    BUN—84520
    Creatinine—82565
    Sodium—84295
    Potassium—84132
    Chloride—82435
    Carbon dioxide—82374
    Calcium—82310

3. Hepatic function panel—80076

    Transferase, aspartate amino (AST)(SGOT)—84450
    Transferase, alanine amino (ALT)(SGPT)—84460
    Phosphatase, alkaline—84075
    Bilirubin, total—82247
    Bilirubin, direct—82248
    Protein, total—84155
    Albumin—82040

4. Acute hepatitis panel—80074

    Hepatitis B surface antigen (HBsAG)—87340
    Hepatitis B core antibody (HbcAb), IgM antibody—86705
    Hepatitis C antibody—86803
    Hepatitis A antibody (HAAb), IgM antibody—86709

5. Renal function panel—80069

    Creatinine—82565
    Urea nitrogen (BUN)—84520
    Calcium—82310
    Phosphorus, inorganic (phosphate)—84100
    Sodium—84295
    Potassium—84132
    Carbon dioxide—82374
    Chloride—82435
    Albumin—82040
    Glucose—82947

6. Electrolyte panel—80051

    Carbon dioxide—82374
    Chloride—82435
    Potassium—84132
    Sodium—84295

patient. Unfortunately the Health Care Financing Administration's concern over test utilization and medical necessity have precluded an expansion of organ-and-disease panels, despite the preference of physicians for the convenience of ordering measurements and examinations in panels. However, anticipated Current Procedural Terminology (CPT) codes in the year 2000 enhance five of the six organ-and-disease panels, as shown in Table 3–2.

Each individual undoubtedly has his or her own more narrow reference interval (normal value) for each measurement that should and can be established over time with repeated measurements adjusted for methodology. An individual's normal value for a particular measurement or test may be 50% or less than the reported reference interval, or normal value.

Risk-factor assessment incorporates such an approach, which can and should be expanded. The potential, powerful strength of laboratory measurements has yet to be implemented fully with data reduction and graphic display over time through a computerized patient record (CPR) or a lifetime medical record. Laboratory measurements and examinations yield the most hard scientific data or information that compose a patient's medical record with recognition that laboratory determinations are not always infallible. With a graphic display and trends evident, measurements in organ panels or disease profiles will be even more valuable and helpful in diagnosis and management.

Over 70% of medical care costs can be attributed to medical decisions based on laboratory measurements and examinations. Thus we owe to our patients and clinicians as well as the public even more cost-effective, efficient, and accessible test menus with the highest quality results that lend themselves to interpretation with trends graphically evident.

4

CONFIRMATION REQUEST AND VALIDATION OF DETERMINATIONS

A confirmation request is a systematic and objective approach to conflict resolution (most often over a test result) between the laboratory staff and a user of clinical laboratory information or data. We have already indicated in Chapter 2 that a laboratory determination result though scientifically accurate and precise may not be perceived as such. In Chapter 3 the last resort in quality assurance (QA) is referred to as the patient's physician or attending physician of record. The user or customer may also be a nurse practitioner (NP) or physician assistant (PA) or someone calling on behalf of an attending. Our clinical colleagues, who are responsible and accountable for a patient's diagnosis and management, must be able to make a good decision on behalf of the patient based on all the information available, clinical experience, and judgment at that time. In Chapter 2 we also indicated that it was acceptable for colleagues to differ in opinions and interpretation.

Medicine is both an art and a science with clinical judgment from experience integrated into our thinking, actions, and decisions. There is every need and reason for a clinician to have confidence in each and every laboratory measurement and examination. If he or she does not have such confidence at a time of need or an impending decision that will modify clinical management or therapy, let alone a diagnosis in the course of a patient's illness or disease (see Fig. 1–1), we in the laboratory have all been remiss in supporting or assisting our clinical colleagues in patient care. Clinicians are not only our most important customers in patient care, but also busy individuals often under great stress in responding to needs and demands of more than one critically ill patient at any one time. There should be no doubt or delay in responding to this situation of potential conflict.

A confirmation request is without charge; it is responsive to a conflict or concern resolution by the clinician, who communicates, preferably in writing, an order for a "confirmation request" indicating the specific measurement or measurements in question, e.g., potassium (K), digoxin level, or even a hematocrit. This is a *stat*. request and is so responded to by laboratory staff in receiving a new specimen with a request form indicating suspected analytes and marked "confirmation request." Laboratorians then retrieve a prior specimen on this patient and promptly repeat determinations on both original and subsequent specimens with reports indicating both results (date and time of each specimen, collection, and analysis), and concluding "confirmed," i.e., within precision or coefficient of variation of the measurement in question, or "unconfirmed." An "unconfirmed" conclusion requires prompt follow-through including checking both specimens for patient identifications, including full name and hospital number, as well as within-run and between-run quality control (QC) values and delta checks for each assay in question. If that does not resolve the question, a third specimen for validation must be obtained and analyzed. Again, this specimen is collected with meticulous attention as to identification of both patient and specimen with performance follow-through of the analyses in the most expeditious manner for all three specimens. Rarely is it necessary to add a third specimen or an additional measurement to confirm a determination in question, e.g., a gamma-glutamyl transpeptidase (GGT) determination to confirm an alkaline phosphatase abnormality in a particular patient's blood.

Indeed, our experience over the years is that such measurements are confirmed expeditiously and conflict is resolved in more than 98% of the times requested. Rarely, errors in patient identification or request forms, specimen-labeling errors, or contamination are precipitating events. With a patient or specimen-identification error, it is equally important to pursue and find the other specimen and correct patient or presumed other patient suspected in receiving a reciprocal, inappropriate laboratory measurement or examination result; this must be resolved in a comparable manner and requires special diligence in pursuit of this discrepancy.

The clinician retains confidence in laboratory information and morale among laboratory personnel is sustained when a confirmation request has been properly and promptly executed, with results returned confirming or validating values. It should never be an issue of "believing in laboratory results." Faith is not a consideration in laboratory information or data, since laboratory results can and should be subjected to hard scientific validation through a confirmation request.

In the end, the patient benefits and clinicians can make the most appropriate decision on behalf of their patient with confidence in the laboratory's performance and continued appreciation and recognition for accurate, reproducible information or data. There should never be a reason for a clinician or any other laboratory customer to doubt the validity of any or several laboratory measurements for any one patient at any time of day or night. A promptly executed "confirmation request" should resolve such issues expeditiously in a definitive, objective manner to benefit all.

COMMON CALLS IN CLINICAL PATHOLOGY FROM WITHIN THE LABORATORY AND OUTSIDE

□ □ □

5

GENERAL PROBLEMS: INSTRUMENTATION, INFORMATION SYSTEMS, AND PERSONNEL

INSTRUMENT PROBLEMS
    Instrument Failure
    Erroneous Results
UNLABELED AND MISLABELED SPECIMENS
PERSONNEL ISSUES

Some general issues affect all sections of clinical pathology and relate to instruments, information systems, and personnel. Several of these are becoming more important as automation in the laboratory increases and the health care payment or reimbursement environment changes.

■ INSTRUMENT PROBLEMS

All laboratory instruments undergo preventive maintenance according to schedules recommended by the manufacturer. In addition, regular calibration and quality control checks help ensure accuracy of the results produced. However, as with all things mechanical, things can and do go wrong from time to time. It is essential to recognize a malfunction at the earliest time, so that erroneous values are not reported.

Instrument Failure

Instrument failures lead to delays in turnaround time and can have serious consequences for patients. Larger laboratories may have backup instruments to which they can switch in case an instrument fails. Another option is to use a different laboratory in the area (for urgent tests) or to send out specimens to a commercial laboratory. In any event, the situation needs to be critically analyzed and potential patient consequences considered.

The pathologist has to work actively with the technical staff for prompt resolution of such problems.

- *Nature of the malfunction.* Experienced technical personnel can usually determine the nature of most malfunctions and correct

them. Instrument manufacturers usually have a 24-hour technical assistance "hotline" and may be able to diagnose the problem and provide a solution over the phone. If delays are expected in reporting results, the pathologist should be informed
and should consider further action. In-hospital clinical engineer-
ing service may be available in some institutions for such re-
pairs, response, and preventive maintenance.

- *Tests affected.* The pathologist needs to consider the clinical effect of
  the expected delays and decide the subsequent course of action.
- *Authorize sendout.* For those tests whose results are required urgently, the specimens should be sent out to another laboratory. This
  requires authorization by the pathologist. The pathologist and
  technical personnel can design a standard operating procedure
  (SOP) for sending out urgent and *stat.* specimens so that unnecessary delays while authorization is being sought can be avoided.
- *Communicate with clinicians.* If test results are expected to be delayed beyond the usual turnaround time, the pathologist should
  let the clinicians know of the expected delays and the steps being taken to address the problem. The pathologist and clinician
  need to consider alternative tests that may help patient care. If
  the clinician indicates that the expected delay would not cause
  adverse patient consequences, the laboratory can avoid unnecessary (and expensive) sendouts.

A retrospective analysis of such situations may reveal a procedural or training lapse that can be corrected. With experienced
personnel and SOPs, adverse patient consequences should not
occur.

Erroneous Results (see also Chapter 3)

Erroneous test results stem from a variety of different problems
that can be divided into three broad groups:

- *Preanalytical* includes test requisition, patient preparation, specimen collection, specimen transport, specimen identification
  (unidentified and mislabeled specimens are discussed in the
  next section).
- *Analytical* includes instrument- or procedure-dependent biases,
  random variability, quality of reagents and supplies, temperature, etc.
- *Postanalytical* includes reporting of results and is influenced by
  the nature of the laboratory information system and the inter-
  face between different instruments and the laboratory and hospital information systems.

The potential for errors is minimized by careful attention to all
steps involved in generating a test result and by the process of

quality control. However, some processes, such as those at the pre-analytical stage, are often outside the control of the laboratory.

If a reported test result is found to be erroneous, a revised report should be issued immediately. In addition, if the error is of major clinical significance, the pathologist should discuss the revised report with the ordering physician and make a note in the patient's medical record. This should include specific recommendations regarding specimen collection and test ordering if that is the source of the problem. Chapter 4 reviews an option in quality assurance as a confirmation request.

■ UNLABELED AND MISLABELED SPECIMENS

Specimens received in the laboratory without appropriate patient identification should not be processed, and a repeat specimen should be requested. It is the responsibility of the individual collecting the specimen to label it appropriately at the time of collection. If the specimen is determined to be one of a kind by the individual responsible for collection, he or she must personally identify the specimen in the laboratory and label it. Such specimens are usually body fluids or tissues that cannot be collected again. In our laboratory, we have a standard form for such specimens (Fig. 5–1). A copy of the form is sent to the risk-management department. The report issued on such specimens includes a statement to the effect that the specimen was received inappropriately labeled and was subsequently identified and labeled by the person who collected it and declared it to be "one of a kind."

The blood bank should not process an unlabeled or mislabeled blood specimen for pretransfusion testing under any circumstances. Unresponsive patients whose identity is unknown should get a temporary identification bracelet, which should be used, usually through and with another person such as a nurse close to the patient for confirmation, until proper identity can be established.

■ PERSONNEL ISSUES

Formerly, we staffed for peak demands in work load. In this era of cost containment, laboratory staffing is usually maintained at the minimum possible. Complex tests, which are usually performed by more experienced technologists, are therefore not available 24 hours a day in most laboratories. A *stat.* request for such a test requires one to call in a technologist who then earns compensatory time off or overtime pay. Laboratories can ill afford overtime pay, and compensatory time off leads to difficulties in scheduling

"ONE OF A KIND" MISLABELED/UNLABELED SPECIMENS

Pathology Laboratory Destination:_____

Date and time received in Lab:_____

Individual contacted concerning unlabeled specimen:_____,
                                                        Name

_____, and _____/_____
          Extension   Date/Time

Test(s) requested on specimen: _____

Accession # _____

Brief description of specimen: (e.g., 2 mL yellow urine in plastic tube):

_____

Reason why repeat specimen cannot be obtained: _____

_____

   I certify that I, (print name)_____ , can identify the
mislabeled/unlabeled specimen, consisting of_____ , which is
described above, and that I collected the specimen from the patient
(name)_____ , (hospital #)_____ , on (day)
_____at (time)_____ . I will appropriately label this specimen.
I understand that the Pathology Laboratory will issue a report with the
results including the statement that this specimen was received mislabeled/
unlabeled and was declared "one of a kind" and then labeled by me.

Signature_____ Date/time_____
Department_____ Extension or beeper #_____

(Mislabeled/unlabeled specimens received by the laboratory and not corrected
by the appropriate personnel cannot be processed.)

cc: Risk Management

Figure 5–1 □ One-of-a-kind specimen form.

and work-load distribution in normal working hours, which has
an adverse effect on turnaround time.

   The pathologist is called on to approve requests for *stat.* tests,
which involve calling in a technologist. It is the pathologist's responsibility to discuss the clinical situation with the ordering

physician and clearly establish the indication for the test. The test result should have an immediate effect on patient care. The pathologist should also secure the telephone or pager number of the ordering physician so that the result can be called in directly to the ordering physician. In many instances it may be possible to delay the test until the next morning and have the technologist perform it early in the day without compromising patient care.

TRANSFUSION MEDICINE

Transfusion medicine (TM) encompasses the blood bank, histocompatibility (HLA) laboratory, progenitor cell laboratory, and parentage testing service in addition to hemapheresis service considered in Chapter 7. TM policies and procedures precede discussion of blood and blood components/derivatives and special blood products; all are a prerequisite for presentation of an effective role of resident on call. Five major topics then extend and expand the role of the resident on call in fulfilling call responsibilities.

■ OVERVIEW: POLICIES AND PROCEDURES

Blood Transfusion Consent

Patients requiring nonemergent transfusion of blood or blood components must have a current, signed Consent to Transfuse form in the medical record (Fig. 6–1). A signed consent form is required for each hospital admission or every 90 days for a single hospital admission. For patients transfused on an outpatient basis, a signed consent form is required once a year. If an outpatient subsequently requires admission to the hospital, a new consent form should be obtained. For surgical procedures, a Consent to Transfuse form should be obtained in all procedures requiring either a "type and screen" or "type and crossmatch." A patient information brochure, such as "If You Need a Blood Transfusion," should be available for patient reading or review. A patient refusing a blood transfusion against the advice of his or her physician must sign a Refusal of Blood Transfusion form (Fig. 6–2).

Specimens for Blood Bank Procedures and Tests

Specimens for blood bank tests must be accompanied by a blood component order form (BCOF). Both the specimen label and the BCOF must include the patient's full name, medical record number, date and time specimen was drawn, and the initials of the phlebotomist (Figs. 6–3 to 6–6). UNLABELED OR MISLABELED SPECIMENS CANNOT BE ACCEPTED, nor should the blood bank recognize "one of a kind" specimens. A new specimen MUST be drawn if a mislabeled or unlabeled specimen is received.

Ordering Blood and Blood Products

A blood component order form (BCOF) is required for all blood-product orders (Figs. 6–3 to 6–6). The BCOF must contain the patient's full name, the medical record number, the type of product ordered, the number of units ordered, and the clinical justification or rationale for transfusion. The form must be signed by the ordering or requesting physician. In an emergency, the form may be signed by a nurse, indicating the name of the ordering physician. The blood bank also needs to be called in advance for orders of fresh frozen plasma, cryoprecipitate, or special blood products (see the later discussions of blood components and special blood products).

Last Name: First Name: MRN: DOB: Patient addressograph or full name and MRN	UNIVERSITY **HOSPITAL** **CONSENT TO TRANSFUSE**

(This form is intended only for use when nonemergency transfusions are anticipated, and it can be used as an alternative or supplement to a physician's transfusion note written in the medical record. Complete this form at the time of diagnosis or at the time major changes in therapy occur.)

Patient Name:_____
Patient Diagnosis/Procedure:_____
Hospitalization or estimated dates of treatment:_____ to_____

During your treatment, you may need transfusions of blood products for the following reasons:

- Anemia (low red cell count), thrombocytopenia (low platelet count), and leukopenia (low white blood cell count) can occur as a result of your disorder or its treatment. Correction of anemia with red cell transfusions, correction of the thrombocytopenia with platelet transfusions, and correction of leukopenia with white blood cell transfusions may be necessary.
- Decreased blood clotting factors can occur as a result of your disorder or its treatment. Replacement of the clotting factors by transfusions of blood plasma products may be necessary.

The risks of blood transfusions are as follows:

- Infections such as hepatitis and HIV (AIDS), which are very infrequent.
- Other complications such as transfusion reactions (fever, anxiety, chills, and discomfort) and changes in immunity may occur, especially if many transfusions are necessary.

I have read and understand the above information, as well as University Hospital's pamphlet "If You Need a Blood Transfusion." My physician has explained the risks and benefits of blood transfusions and answered my questions. I agree to allow authorized members of the hospital staff to give me blood transfusions when deemed medically necessary.

_____   _____
Date   Time   Signature of Patient or Guardian

Figure 6–1 □ Blood transfusion consent form. See p. 53 for transfusion-transmitted diseases and p. 88 for transfusion reactions.

Refusal of Blood Transfusion

The dangers of not proceeding with the recommended transfusion have been explained to me. Risks of not receiving a transfusion may include uncontrollable bleeding, anemia, organ failure, and death.

I personally assume the risks and consequences of refusal to consent to the transfusion(s), and I release all physicians who have been consulted in my case, the hospital, and its staff from liability and damages for any ill effects that may result from not being transfused.

I have read this entire document, and I understand its contents. In addition, I have completed or crossed off any unacceptable statements before my signing.

I <u>do not</u> consent to receive blood transfusions.

Date   Time   Signature of Patient or Guardian

Witness:

Date   Time   Signature of Witness

Physician: I have discussed the treatment described above with the patient or relative whose signature appears on this document.

Date   Time   Signature of Physician

CROSS OUT ANY OF THE ABOVE PARAGRAPHS THAT DO NOT APPLY AND INITIAL.

Figure 6–2 □ Refusal of blood transfusion form.

Returning Blood and Blood Components

Unopened units may be returned to the blood bank within 30 minutes of issue. If opened or delayed over 30 minutes, the unit will be discarded.

Monitored Refrigerators

Blood may be stored only in monitored refrigerators located in selected areas such as the Emergency Medicine Department, Recovery Room, and Cardiopulmonary Surgical Intensive Care Unit. BLOOD SHOULD NOT BE PLACED IN UNMONITORED REFRIGERATORS ON NURSING UNITS. Storage of blood in un-

Location: | University **Hospital** RBC

Patient addressograph or full name and Medical Record # | Department of Clinical Pathology
RBC ORDER FORM

| Diagnosis | Collected by:
Date/Time Collected |

☐ Routine (4 hr) ☐ Type & Screen   Date & Time of Transfusion: _____
☐ Expedite (2 hr) ☐ Type & Crossmatch   Date & Time of Surgery: _____
☐ Stat (1 hr)   Surgical Procedure: _____

| No. Component
Required Desired | No. Component
Required Desired | Special Needs |

__ Red Blood Cells   __ Leukoreduced red cells   __ CMV negative product required
__ Irradiated red cells   __ Irradiated leukoreduced red cells   __ Split red cell required (advance
__ Washed red cells   __ Frozen deglycerolized red cells   call required for preparation)
__ Directed donor red cells   __ Autologous red cells

III. PLEASE MARK ALL APPROPRIATE BOXES: Hct: _____ Time: _____ Date: _____
☐ Pre Op orders
☐ Hct <21%

☐ Hct 21-30% and one or more boxes in Column A **AND** in Column B

A. Risk of myocardial or cerebral ischemia | B. Physiological evidence that the patient needs more hemoglobin
☐ Patient at risk for myocardial ischemia   ☐ Active bleeding, site: _____
☐ Coronary artery disease   ☐ During surgery: _____
☐ Valvular heart disease   ☐ Rapidly falling hematocrit
☐ Congestive heart failure   ☐ Syncope
☐ Patient at risk for cerebral ischemia   ☐ Dyspnea
☐ History of transient ischemic attacks   ☐ Postural hypotension
☐ Previous thrombotic stroke   ☐ Oliguria
☐ Coagulopathy   ☐ Tachycardia
☐ Outpatient   ☐ Angina
  ☐ Transient ischemic attack

☐ Hct >30% and invasively monitored patient with supply dependent O_2 consumption
  (O_2 consumption [VO_2] increasing with increased O_2 transport [DO_2])
☐ Maintenance therapy for chronic anemia such as thalassemia
☐ Pre-op Hct <33.0% in sickle cell patient
☐ Patient on chemotherapy
☐ Special circumstance

IV. **NOTE:** These are gidelines for blood transfusion practice. If the clinical situation is outside these guidelines, or if adverse effects are associated with the use of these guidelines, please contact the Blood Bank for physician consultation.

Ordering Physician: _____ MD/DO   Beeper: _____
(PLEASE PRINT OR STAMP)

Physician's Signature: _____ MD/DO   Date: _____ Time: _____
(REQUIRED)

Nurse's Signature: _____ RN   Date: _____ Time: _____
(IN EMERGENCY)

Blood Bank Use: _____
41430 – RBC Order Form – Rev. 5/97 WHITE – Medical Record YELLOW – Blood Bank PINK – Bring to Blood Bank Pick-up Product G3.00

Figure 6–3 ☐ Red blood cell order form.

			University **Hospital**
			Department of Clinical Pathology **FFP & CRYOPRECIPITATE**
Patient addressograph or full name and Medical Record #			**ORDER FORM**

I. UNIT:	☐ STAT (1 hr)	☐ EXPEDITE (2 hr):	DATE & TIME FOR TRANSFUSION: _____
DATE:		☐ ROUTINE (4 hr):	DATE & TIME FOR SURGERY: _____

II. FFP: Please mark one or more boxes in Column A **AND** in Column B, **OR** one box in Column C
No. of units requested:_____

COLUMN A
☐ PT > 17 sec
  PT:_____ Time:_____
☐ PTT > 44 sec
  PTT:_____ Time:_____
☐ Active bleeding with coag
  studies pending
☐ DIC, Fib:_____
  or FSP:_____
☐ Severe liver disease

☐ Previously diagnosed
  deficiency of factor:_____
☐ Need to reverse warfarin
  effect
☐ Trauma

COLUMN B
☐ Active bleeding
☐ Prior to or during surgery:
  _____
☐ Prior to invasive procedure:
  _____

COLUMN C
NOTE: Pharmacy has antithrombin III concentrate.
☐ Heparin cofactor II
  deficiency
☐ Protein S deficiency
☐ Protein C deficiency
☐ Post bypass with
  microvascular bleeding
☐ L-asparaginase therapy
  with risk of thrombosis
  due to low Protein C level
  (Keep Fibrinogen > 100 mg/dL)

☐ Special circumstance
  _____
  _____

III. CRYOPRECIPITATE: For von Willebrand's Disease consider Humate P or Alphanate SD from Pharmacy.
Dose: 1 bag/7 kg — No. requested: _____
Please mark appropriate boxes
☐ Bleeding with fibrinogen less than 100 mg/dL
☐ Uremia with platelet dysfunction (Cr ≥5 mg/dL)
☐ Special circumstance_____

IV. NOTE: Prolonged PT and/or PTT values may reflect a lupus anticoagulant rather than a true factor deficiency.
These are not criteria for blood transfusion practice; they are criteria for the review of blood product orders. To
quicken the process, the Clinical Resident should contact the Blood Bank Resident if the clinical situation is outside
these guidelines, or if adverse effects are associated with the use of these guidelines

Ordering Physician:_____ MD/DO   Beeper:_____
                    (PLEASE PRINT OR STAMP)

Physician's Signature:_____ MD/DO   Date:_____ Time:_____
                         (REQUIRED)

Nurse's Signature:_____ RN   Date:_____ Time:_____
                    (IN EMERGENCY)

Blood Bank Use:_____
40885 – FFP & CRYO Order Form – 6/96   WHITE – Medical Record   YELLOW – Blood Bank   G3.00

Figure 6–4 ☐ Fresh frozen plasma and cryoprecipitate order form.

monitored refrigerators may result in bacterial contamination,
freezing, and hemolysis.

Blood for Emergency Transfusion

A specimen sample for a type and crossmatch should be immediately drawn and sent to the blood bank for *stat.* ABO/Rh typing.

University **Hospital**

Department of Clinical Pathology
PLATELET ORDER FORM

Patient addressograph or full name and Medical Record #

I. UNIT:	☐ STAT (1 hr)	☐ EXPEDITE (2 hr):	DATE & TIME FOR TRANSFUSION:_____
DATE:		☐ ROUTINE (4 hr):	DATE & TIME FOR SURGERY:_____

II. NO. REQUESTED:_____

Adult dose: 6 pooled platelet conc
Pediatric dose: 0.2 units/kg pooled platelet conc

TYPE OF PLATELET PRODUCT:

☐ Pooled platelets   ☐ HLA matched
☐ Leukocyte reduced   ☐ Directed donation
☐ Irradiated   ☐ _____
☐ Apheresis/single donor

III. PLEASE MARK APPROPRIATE BOXES: Platelet count:_____   Time:_____   Date:_____

☐ Plt ≤10,000

☐ Plt 11,000   **AND**   Any of Items 1 – 22
to 20,000
- ☐ 1. Rapidly decreasing Plt count   ☐ 7. Heparin or warfarin therapy
- ☐ 2. Severe infection   ☐ 8. Antithymocyte therapy
- ☐ 3. Outpatient   ☐ 9. Malignant melanoma
- ☐ 4. Coagulation defect: ☐ 10. Renal cell carcinoma
- ☐ 5. Uremia (Cr ≥5.0 mg/dL) Cr:__   ☐ 11. Brain lesion
- ☐ 6. History of significant bleeding   ☐ 12. Induction chemotherapy with high WBC

☐ Plt 21,000   **AND**   Any of Items 13 – 22
to 50,000
- ☐ 13. Active bleeding, site:_____
- ☐ 14. Surgery, or invasive procedure planned:_____
- ☐ 15. DIC, FIB:_____ or FSP:_____
- ☐ 16. Plt dysfunction, suspected cause:_____
- ☐ 17. Trauma
- ☐ 18. Prior CNS irradiation

☐ Plt 51,000   **AND**   Any of Items 19 – 22
to 100,000
- ☐ 19. Uncontrollable bleeding, site:_____
- ☐ 20. During surgery for brain, eye, airway:_____
- ☐ 21. Post bypass with chest tube drainage >200 mL/hr., or > 3 mL/kg/hr, drainage:
- ☐ 22. Microvascular bleeding (operative oozing)

☐ Special circumstance:_____

IV. **NOTE:** These are not criteria for blood transfusion practice; they are criteria for the review of blood product orders. To quicken the process, the Clinical Resident should contact the Blood Bank Resident if the clinical situation is outside these guidelines, or if adverse effects are associated with the use of these guidelines

Ordering Physician:_____ MD/DO   Beeper:_____
(PLEASE PRINT OR STAMP)

Physician's Signature:_____ MD/DO   Date:_____ Time:_____
(REQUIRED)

Nurse's Signature:_____ RN   Date:_____ Time:_____
(IN EMERGENCY)

Blood Bank Use:_____
41305 – Platelet Order Form – 5/96   WHITE – Medical Record   YELLOW – Blood Bank   G3.00

Figure 6–5 ☐ Platelet order form.

Uncrossmatched, ABO/Rh type-specific blood should be available within 10 to 15 minutes after a blood specimen is received. Release of uncrossmatched blood requires a signed release statement by the ordering physician. Compatibility testing will then be com-

			University **Hospital**
			Department of Clinical Pathology **ALBUMIN ORDER FORM**

Patient addressograph or full name and Medical Record #

I. UNIT:	☐ STAT (1 hr)	☐ EXPEDITE (2 hr):	DATE & TIME FOR TRANSFUSION: _____
DATE:		☐ ROUTINE (4 hr):	DATE & TIME FOR SURGERY: _____

II. **INFORMATION:** PRIOR TO USING ALBUMIN FOR THE FOLLOWING CONDITIONS, CONSIDER FIRST OR SECOND LINE THERAPY BELOW:

–HYPOVOLEMIA   –BURN PATIENT LESS THAN 24 HOURS AFTER BURN OCCURRED
–HYPOTENSION   –CIRRHOSIS AND PARACENTESIS OF LESS THAN 4 LITERS OF ASCITIC FLUID

FIRST LINE THERAPY	**SECOND LINE THERAPY**
Normal Saline Lactated Ringer's Solution	Hetastarch (Hespan) 6% in NS 500 mL, up to 20 mL/kg/24 hr

III. ALBUMIN: Please mark one or more boxes in column A **AND** in column B, **OR** one box in column C:
No. requested: _____ 250 mL (5%) bottles; _____ 50 mL (25%) vials

COLUMN A
☐ Hypovolemia
☐ Hypotension
☐ Burn patient over 24 hours since burn occurred

COLUMN B
☐ 20-50 mL/kg crystalloid and 20 mL/kg/24 hr hetastarch (Hespan) already given
☐ 20-50 mL/kg crystalloid given and any of the following:
  ☐ Child
  ☐ Previous hypersensitivity to hetastarch
  ☐ Underlying bleeding disorder

COLUMN C
☐ Up to 24 hours post-op
☐ Nephrotic syndrome (with use of a diuretic)
☐ Cirrhosis and paracentesis of 4 L or more of ascitic fluid (in an adult) and albumin <2.5 g/dL.
☐ Plasmapheresis/Plasma Exchange
☐ Severe necrotizing pancreatitis
☐ Hemodialysis with fluid overload, hypotension or unstable cardiovascular status
☐ Hyperbilirubinemia of the newborn (with RBC transfusion)
☐ Pancreas transplant recipient receiving antithymocyte therapy
☐ Significant diarrhea (2 L per day) and serum albumin <3.0 g/dL.
☐ Special circumstance: _____
_____
_____

IV. **NOTE:** These are not criteria for blood transfusion practice; they are criteria for the review of blood product orders. To quicken the process, the Clinical Resident should contact the Blood Bank Resident if the clinical situation is outside these guidelines, or if adverse effects are associated with the use of these guidelines

Ordering Physician: _____ MD/DO   Beeper: _____
     (PLEASE PRINT OR STAMP)

Physician's Signature: _____ MD/DO   Date: _____ Time: _____
     (REQUIRED)

Nurse's Signature: _____ RN   Date: _____ Time: _____
     (IN EMERGENCY)

Blood Bank Use: _____

40028 – Albumin Order Form – 6/96   WHITE – Medical Record   YELLOW – Blood Bank   G3.00

Figure 6–6 ☐ Albumin order form.

pleted and results reported *stat.* if an incompatibility is detected after release of blood.

A protocol for switching ABO blood types, when the patient's type is not available in stock inventory, is shown in Table 6–1.

Table 6–1 □ PROTOCOL FOR SWITCHING BLOOD TYPES

Switching ABO Types

Patients should be transfused with red cell products with the same ABO and Rh type as their own. If ABO type specific red cells are not available, the following list should be used to select ABO compatible blood:

Patient and ABO/Rh	First Choice	First Alternative	Second Alternative	Third Alternative
O Pos	O Pos	None	None	None
A Pos	A Pos	O Pos PC	None	None
B Pos	B Pos	O Pos PC	None	None
AB Pos	AB Pos	A Pos PC	B Pos PC	O Pos PC

Switching Rh Types

Rh-positive recipients can be given Rh-negative units if necessary.

Rh-Negative Recipients <u>Should Not</u> Be Given Rh-Positive Red Cells.

In an emergency, if there are no Rh-negative red cell units available, contact the resident or attending who will then speak with the ordering physician and assess the patient's condition and determine how much blood is needed. If transfusion can be delayed, it should be until Rh-negative units can be obtained. If the patient must be transfused, the resident or attending will advise the ordering physician that we are switching to Rh-positive red cells and of the risks. If a resident or attending cannot be reached, notify the ordering physician directly.

Give Only Rh-Positive in an Emergency.

O Neg (male/female over 45)	O Neg	O Pos PC	None	None
O Neg (female under 45)	O Neg	O Pos PC	None	None
A Neg (male/female over 45)	A Neg	A Pos PC	O Pos PC	None
A Neg (female under 45)	A Neg	O Neg PC	A Pos PC	O Pos PC
B Neg (male/female over 45)	B Neg	B Pos PC	O Pos PC	None
B Neg (female under 45)	B Neg	O Neg PC	B Pos PC	O Pos PC
AB Neg (male/female over 45)	AB Neg	AB Pos PC	A Pos PC B Pos PC	O Pos PC
AB Neg (female under 45)	AB Neg	A Neg PC B Neg PC	O Neg PC	AB Pos PC A Pos PC B Pos PC O Pos PC

In extreme situations, **uncrossmatched group O, Rh_0 (D)-negative red blood cell units** may be released *pending ABO/Rh typing*. Transfusion of uncrossmatched, group O, Rh_0 (D)-negative red cells requires a signed release statement by the ordering physician. It is then imperative that a patient's blood specimen, or sample, for type and crossmatch *stat.*, be sent as soon as possible to the blood bank. Transfusion of group O, Rh_0 (D)-negative red cells with isoagglutinins in plasma may interfere with ABO/Rh typing, and a patient with an alloantibody may experience a hemolytic transfusion reaction when universal donor (O-negative) unit of blood contains the corresponding antigen.

In acute emergencies, the supply of Rh_0 (D)-negative blood may become exhausted. It may be necessary to transfuse Rh_0 (D)-positive blood to an Rh_0 (D)-negative patient. The decision to switch from Rh_0 (D)-negative to Rh_0 (D)-positive blood should be determined by the Transfusion Medicine attending or physician based on local or regional availability of Rh_0 (D)-negative blood units, clinical information on the patient and concurrent or anticipated other patient needs (see Table 6–1).

Massive Transfusion

A massive transfusion occurs when a patient has bled more than one blood volume or experienced a blood loss of approximately 5 liters in 24 hours (for an average 70-kg adult). Most cases of massive transfusion are in the operating room, emergency department, or intensive care settings. The blood bank should automatically contact the pathology resident on call for any adult patient requiring more than 10 units of packed red cells or a child requiring more than 5 units of packed red cells within the previous 24 hours. The pathologist on call will review recent laboratory tests (PT, PTT, fibrinogen, TT, platelet count, hematocrit) and the total number of blood products dispensed and transfused. If the patient is at risk for or shows evidence of a dilutional coagulopathy, the pathologist on call will consult the attending clinician with regard to additional blood product support and laboratory monitoring (p. 81).

Guidelines for Ordering Blood for Elective Surgery

Guidelines for ordering blood to be used in elective surgery have been established (Table 6–2). Orders in excess of the guidelines should be referred to the resident or pathologist on call. The resident will contact the clinician or physician for additional information to ascertain the patient's needs further. Exceptions to guidelines, i.e., anemia or more complex surgery anticipated, can then be made, or the physician may be educated accordingly.

Table 6–2 □ GUIDELINES FOR ORDERING BLOOD FOR ELECTIVE SURGERY

Cardiothoracic

Angioplasty	T&S
Aortic or ventricular aneurysm repair	4
Aortic dissection	6
B.T. shunt	1
Bidirectional Glenn shunt	2
Closure of patent ductus arteriosis	T&S
Coarctation repair	3
Esophagogastrectomy	2
Esophageal hernia	T&S
Esophagoscopy	0
Fontan procedure	3
Great vessel switch	3
Lobectomy	1
Mediastinoscopy	0
Open heart procedures:	
Adult	3
Pediatric	3
Open lung biopsy	T&S
Pacemaker insertion	0
PDA ligation	T&S
Pericardectomy	2
Pericardial window	0
Pneumonectomy	2
Pulmonary valvulotomy	3
Redo and repair	6
Septectomy	2
Sternal wire removal	0
Thoracotomy	2
Thoracoscopy	0
Wedge resection	T&S

General Surgery

Abdominal-perineal resection	2
Amputations	T&S
Appendectomy	0
Bronchoscopy	0
Catheter insertion/removal (Hickman, Life Port Tenkoff, Infuse-a-port)	0
Cholecystojejunostomy	T&S
Cholecystectomy	T&S
Colon resection	T&S
Colostomy closure/ takedown	T&S
Débridement (wound, burn)	AO

Denver peritoneal shunt insertion	0
Denver shunt revision	0
Dressing change	0
Exploratory laparotomy	2
Gastric bypass	T&S
Gastrostomy tube insertion	0
Hemicolectomy	2
Hemorrhoidectomy	0
Hepatic lobectomy	6
Hernia repair, incisional Inguinal, (inguinal herniorrhaphy)	0
Ileostomy	T&S
Iliac profunda bypass	1
Jejunostomy tube placement	0
Lumpectomy, breast mass excision	0
Mastectomy:	
Simple	0
Modified, radical	T&S
Mediastinoscopy	0
Myotomy (pyloric)	0
Oophorectomy	T&S
Parotidectomy	T&S
Pilonidal cyst	0
Porto-caval shunt	4
Pseudo-aneurysm repair	6
Rib resection	0
Sigmoidectomy	T&S
Sigmoidoscopy	0
Small bowel resection	T&S
Splenectomy	T&S
Sympathectomy	T&S
Thyroidectomy:	
Parathyroidectomy	0
Partial, total	0
Total large colon resection	T&S
Tracheostomy	0-T&S
Vagotomy	0
Vein stripping	T&S
Whipple procedure	2

Gynecology

AP repair	1
Cone biopsy (CO_2 laser)	0
D&C	0
Ectopic pregnancy	2

Table continued on following page

Table 6–2 □ **GUIDELINES FOR ORDERING BLOOD FOR ELECTIVE SURGERY** *Continued*

Gynecology *Continued*		Orthopedics	
Endometrium ablation	0	Acromioplasty	0
Examination under anesthesia (EUA)	0	Amputation	T&S
		Arthroscopy	0
Exploratory laparotomy	T&S-2	Arthroplasty	T&S
Exteneration procedure	4	Arthrotomy	0
Hysterectomy, total abdominal	T&S-2	Biopsy, excisional	0
		Bipolar transfer	T&S
Hysteroscopy	0	Carpal tunnel release	0
Groshong catheter insertion	0	Closed reduction	0
		Débridement	A0
Laparoscopy	0	Decompression laminectomy	T&S
Laser vaporization	0	Discectomy	T&S
Neosalpingostomy	T&S	Fractures	0
Ovarian wedge resection	T&S	Fusions, other	1
Salpingo- and oophorectomy	0	Hardware removal	0
		Hip revision	3
Uterine suspension	0	Hip screw and nailing	T&S
Tubal ligation	0	Lumbar laminectomy	T&S
Tuboplasty	T&S	Meniscectomy	0
Vaginectomy	T&S	Nerve transposition	0
Vulvectomy	T&S	Neuroma excision	0
		Open reduction	T&S
Neurosurgery		Osteotomy	0
Aneurysm clipping	6	Posterior rod fusion	2
Biopsy (cervical/brain)	T&S-1	Prosthesis removal	T&S
Burr hole	T&S	Releases	0
Carpal tunnel release	0	Revascularization and exploration	T&S
Cervical decompression	T&S-2		
Cervical discectomy	T&S	Rodding (Grosse & Kempf)	T&S
Cordotomy	T&S		
Cordectomy	1	Rotator cuff repair	T&S
Craniectomy	2	Shoulder replacement	T&S
Cranioplasty	T&S	Shoulder repair	0
Craniotomy	2	Spinal fusions	1
Hypophysectomy	T&S-1	Tendon repair	0
Laminectomy	T&S-2	Total elbow	T&S
Lobectomy	2	Total hip	2
Neuroma removal	T&S	Total knee	T&S
Nerve repair	T&S		
Pituitary tumor resection	1	**Otolaryngology (ENT)**	
Spinal fusion	1	Antrotomy	0
Stereotaxis procedure; brain biopsy	T&S	Atticoantrotomy	0
		Bronchoscopy	0
Stereotaxis procedure; hematoma	T&S	Caldwell-Luc	T&S
		Cochlear implant	0
Ulnar nerve transplant	0	Composite resection	4
VP shunt insertion	T&S		

Table 6–2 □ GUIDELINES FOR ORDERING BLOOD FOR ELECTIVE SURGERY *Continued*

Otolaryngology (ENT) *Continued*

Dissecting laryngoscopy	0
Endoscopy	0
Esophageal reconstruction	T&S
Esophagoscopy	0
Ethmoid artery ligation	4
Ethmoidectomy	T&S
Excisional biopsy	0
Frontal sinus, exploration	T&S
Glossectomy	T&S
Labyrinthectomy	0
Laryngectomy	1
Laryngoscopy	0
Mandibulectomy	T&S
Mastoidectomy	T&S
Maxillary fixation	T&S
Maxillectomy	2
Myringotomy	0
Nasopharyngoscopy	0
Neck dissection	2
Neurectomy	0-T&S
Panendoscopy	0-T&S
Parotidectomy	0-T&S
Plate removal	0
Septoplasty	0-T&S
Septorhinoplasty	0-T&S
Sphenoethmoidectomy	T&S
Sphenoidectomy	T&S
Stapedectomy	0
Thyroidectomy	0
Tonsillectomy	0
Tracheoscopy	0
Tracheostomy tube insertion	0
Tracheotomy	T&S
Tympanomastoidectomy	0-T&S
Tympanoplasty	0

Plastic Surgery

Millard repair	T&S
Orbitotomy	T&S
Septorhinoplasty	0-T&S

Transplantation

AV fistula	0
Donor nephrectomy	T&S
Pancreas transplant (leukoreduced)	4
Permanent vascular Catheter insertion/ Removal (Tenckhoff)	0
Renal artery-vein patch	3
Renal transplant (recipient) (leukoreduced products)	2

Urology

Adrenalectomy	2
Bladder resection	T&S
Circumcision	0
Cystectomy	2
Cystoscopy	0
Cystotomy	T&S
Fulguration, bleeding bladder	0
Hydrocelectomy	
Ileal conduit	1
Lithotomy, utero-	T&S
Lithotripsy, shock wave	0
Meatotomy	T&S
Needle biopsy of prostate	0
Nephrectomy, donor	1
Nephrectomy, radical	2
Nephrolithotripsy	1
Nephrostomy	T&S
Orchiopexy	0
Orchiectomy	0
Penectomy	2
Penile prosthesis insertion	0
Prostatectomy	1
Pyelolithotomy	T&S
Reimplantation of ureter	T&S
Stamey procedure	0-T&S
TUR	T&S
Ureterectomy	0
Ureterolithotomy	T&S
Ureteroscopy	0
Urethral fistulas, excision	T&S
Vasectomy	0
Vasovasostomy	0

Vascular Surgery

Abdominal/aortic surgery	2
Aneurysm repair	2
AV fistula	0

Table continued on following page

Table 6–2 □ GUIDELINES FOR ORDERING BLOOD
FOR ELECTIVE SURGERY *Continued*

Vascular Surgery *Continued*		Permanent vascular renal	3
Carotid endarterectomy	T&S	artery repair	
Catheter insertion/removal	0	Splenorenal artery bypass	T&S
Femoral bypass	T&S		
Iliac profunda bypass	1		

Key

1. 0—no work done if specimen received during preadmission testing or blood is drawn when patient is admitted. If no specimen is received Blood Bank will not call the floor to request sample. If work is needed, floor must call to request T&S or crossmatch.
2. T&S—ABO/Rh and antibody screen performed. If no specimen received, Blood Bank will call and notify floor.
3. #Units—this number of units automatically set up. If no specimen received, Blood Bank will call and notify floor.
4. If more units are requested than indicated on this schedule, a technologist or resident will call the physician to determine why additional units are needed. AO means 'as ordered'.
5. Autologous blood—if the patient has donated blood, these units will be crossmatched even if the procedure requires only a type and screen. If the patient donates more units than indicated on this schedule, all units will be crossmatched. If a mixture of autologous and homologous units are set up to meet the patient's surgical needs, only the autologous units will be taken to the OR.

In general, a type and screen (T&S) is appropriate when the likelihood of blood transfusion is less then 10%, i.e., selected elective operations (see Table 6–2). If a transfusion is subsequently required, a T&S can be converted quickly to a type and crossmatch. An electronic crossmatch environment will eventually modify this response.

Transfusion Reaction Evaluation

Suspected transfusion reactions should be reported to the blood bank promptly. The transfusion reaction evaluation standard operating procedure (SOP) is as follows:

Method   ABO/Rh type of pretransfusion and posttransfusion specimens, direct antiglobulin test, visual inspection of serum for hemolysis, posttransfusion urine for hemoglobin, and clerical check on all work performed. Additional testing is performed based on the findings of the initial tests performed.

Specimen	After transfusion: 7 mL of blood, red, plain; 5 mL of whole blood in Versene (lavender, EDTA) tube, and 10 mL of urine.
Transport	Room temperature
Collection	Transfusion reaction form (Fig. 6–7) requisition. Specimens and form must have patient's full name, medical record number, date, and initials of phlebotomist.
TAT (turnaround time)	Daily
Interpretation	Data from tests used to determine if an immediate intravascular hemolytic reaction has occurred. A final written interpretation will be provided after evaluation of all laboratory and clinical findings by resident and attending pathologist (Fig. 6–7; for further information see p. 88 discussing transfusion reactions).

Review of Blood Transfusion: Needs, Benefits, and Risks

Over 4 million Americans receive blood transfusions each year. Blood is used to save the lives of patients who need surgery or other medical treatment, for accident victims, and for patients with cancer, hemophilia, and other serious diseases.

Blood products are shown in Tables 6–3 and 6–4:

- *Red blood cells,* given to support blood oxygen levels and hemoperfusion.
- *Platelets,* needed for some bleeding problems.
- *Fresh frozen plasma (thawed) with or without concentrated forms of plasma,* needed for some bleeding problems.
- *White blood cells,* given only rarely in special circumstances.
- *Albumin,* 5% or 25% for volume depletion.

Transfusion Benefits and Risks

The benefits may include:

- increasing the amount of oxygen circulating in blood (RBC hemoglobin of 1 g = 1.34 mL of O_2 transport) to support body functions through hemoperfusion.
- replacing factors or cell products in the blood to help stop bleeding.
- replacing blood that may be lost because of bleeding, surgery, or a treatment procedure that may cause red blood cells to be decreased for a time period, **OR**
- other reasons to be explained, e.g., intravascular volume depletion and tissue perfusion.

UNIVERSITY HOSPITAL
BLOOD BANK/TRANSFUSION MEDICINE
TRANSFUSION REACTION EVALUATION

All information must be completed to facilitate prompt laboratory evaluation

Date_____ Time Blood Bank notified of reaction_____ (ext. 46700)
Blood unit number_____ Component transfused: ☐ Red cells ☐ Platelets ☐ Plasma ☐ Cryoprecipitate
Time transfusion initiated_____ Time terminated_____ Amount of product transfused_____ mL

BEDSIDE CLERICAL CHECK: Did patient wristband information match that on the transfusion tag? ☐ Yes ☐ No

Vital signs: Blood pressure   Before transfusion_____ At time transfusion was terminated_____
             Body temperature Before transfusion_____ At time transfusion was terminated_____
             Pulse   Before transfusion_____ At time transfusion was terminated_____

Symptoms/Signs Present: (Check all that apply)
☐ Chills ☐ Fever ☐ Chest pain ☐ Shortness of breath ☐ Back pain ☐ Hypotension ☐ Hemoglobinuria
☐ Nausea ☐ Flushing ☐ Hives/Rash ☐ Wheezing   ☐ Headache ☐ Hypertension ☐ Tachycardia

_____ Nurse signature

Other Clinical Findings and Assessment:

_____ MD

INITIAL EVALUATION

Clerical check performed: All information on specimens, requisitions, and donor units correct: ☐ Yes ☐ No
Hemolysis Check: Free Hgb in post-trans. serum _____ Free hgb in post-trans. urine_____
Free hgb in pre-trans. serum _____

	ABO Grouping				Rh Typing			Recipient DAT			
	Anti-A	Anti-B	A1 Cells	B Cells	Anti-D	D Control	AHG	Anti-IgG	Anti-C3	Pos. Cont.	Interpretation
Recipient's pre-transfusion specimen											
Recipient's post-transfusion specimen											
Unit no. (segment/aliquot)			▨	▨			▨	▨	▨	▨	

☐ No further work indicated

| | Screening for Irregular Antibodies | | | | | Crossmatch with Bag | | | | |
	37 C		AHG			Segment or Aliquot				
	SI	SII	SI	SII	Pos. Cont.	I.S.	37 C	AHG	Pos. Cont.	Interpretation
Recipient's pre-transfusion specimen										
Recipient's post-transfusion specimen										

_____ Blood Bank Technologist

OTHER EXAMINATIONS/MEASUREMENTS:
Gram stain on blood bag: Culture on residual:

CLINICAL IMPRESSION & FOLLOW-UP: (Please see reverse)   C24.00 - Rev 11/97

Figure 6–7A ☐ Transfusion reaction evaluation form (obverse side).

Figure 6–7B □ Transfusion reaction evaluation form (reverse side).

Table 6–3 □ COMMON BLOOD COMPONENTS AND DERIVATIVES USED IN HEMOTHERAPY

Blood Component or Derivative	Characteristics	Approximate Volume	Shelf Life	Indications and Comments
Whole blood	RBC and plasma; WBC and platelets not viable after 24 hr storage. Labile clotting factors significantly decreased after 2 days of storage. Hct 35% (dilution by anticoagulant). Blood 450 mL, CPD or CPDA-1 anticoagulant 63 mL.	520 mL	ACD, CPD—21 days at 1–6°C. CPDA-1—35 days at 1–6°C.	Most useful for massive transfusion where both red cell mass and plasma volume are required; active, brisk bleeding. The flow characteristics are rapid. Whole blood is rarely used and generally unavailable.
Packed red blood cells	Packed RBC with reduced plasma volume; WBC, platelets, and coagulation factors as for whole blood. Hct 69%	260 mL	As whole blood.	Most useful for increasing red cell mass when symptomatic anemia is present; chronic anemia. Hct is high, so flow characteristics are viscous and slow. Can be used with colloids or crystalloids to increase rate of flow for active, brisk bleeding or massive transfusion.
Red blood cells with additive solution (adenine-saline)	RBC with reduced plasma volume and an additional 100 mL of additive solution. Hct 53%	340 mL	42 days at 1–6°C.	Can be used like whole blood or packed red blood cells. Hct is at a slightly elevated level but rapid flow rates can be achieved.

Component	Composition	Volume	Storage	Indications/Comments
Washed red blood cells	RBC, no plasma, minimal platelets. 70–80% WBC removed if manual wash. 90% WBC removed if automated wash. Hct adjustment as per amount of saline added. 5% loss of red cells due to wash procedure.	250 mL	24 hr at 1–6°C after wash.	Increased red cell mass as for packed red cells. Most useful for preventing febrile and allergic reactions due to leukocytes or plasma proteins and for preventing anaphylactic reaction in IgA-deficient recipients.
Frozen deglycerolized red blood cells	RBC, no plasma, no platelets, removal of 95% of WBC. Hct adjustment as per amount of saline added. Up to 20% of red cells lost due to procedure.	250 mL	10 years at −65°C or colder. 24 hr at 1–6°C after wash.	Most useful for supply of rare blood, inventory control, and autotransfusion. Also, as per washed red blood cells.
Random-donor platelet concentrate	Platelets (5.5×10^{10}); some WBC (i.e., lymphocytes), 50 mL of plasma, for RBC (less than 0.5% Hct).	50 mL	5 days, room temperature (20–24°C) constant, gentle agitation.	Used for quantitative or qualitative platelet disorders. May be used when bleeding (slow ooze) due to severe thrombocytopenia or for prophylactic therapy. 6–10 units raises platelet count about 50,000 per microliter in adult.
Single-donor platelet concentrate by apheresis	Platelets (3.0×10^{11}); some WBC (i.e., lymphocytes), 250 mL plasma, few RBCs (less than 0.5% Hct).	250 to 300 mL	5 days at room temperature, constant, gentle agitation, 1 day if open system.	Indications as per random-donor platelets. Used as supplement to inventory when there are not enough random-donor platelets. Most useful in immunologically refractory patient when given as HLA match with recipient. Fewer donor exposures.

Table continued on following page

Table 6-3 □ COMMON BLOOD COMPONENTS AND DERIVATIVES USED IN HEMOTHERAPY *Continued*

Blood Component or Derivative	Characteristics	Approximate Volume	Shelf Life	Indications and Comments
Single-donor granulocyte concentrate by apheresis	Granulocytes (1.0×10^{10}) and other WBC, 250 mL plasma, minimal platelets, RBC about 10% Hct.	300 mL	12–24 hr at room temperature, no agitation.	Most useful for septic, severely granulocytopenic patient unresponsive to 48 hr of antibiotic therapy. Potential for aggregated WBC to plug pulmonary capillaries. Perform RBC crossmatch because of quantity of RBC present.
Fresh frozen plasma	Plasma proteins, all coagulation factors, complement.	200 to 260 mL	1 year at −18°C, or colder.	Most useful in the bleeding patient with multiple coagulation deficiency problems secondary to liver disease, disseminated intravascular coagulopathy (DIC), or dilutional changes from massive transfusions. Also useful for the treatment of factor V or factor XI deficiency. Should not be used as volume expander or source of protein nutrition because of risk of transfusion-transmitted disease.

Cryoprecipitate	80 units of factor VIII, other plasma proteins, von Willebrand factor, factor XIII, fibrinogen (200 mg), fibronectin.	10 to 15 mL	1 year at −18°C or colder.	Most useful for von Willebrand disease, factor XIII deficiency, or hypofibrinogenemia. See text for exception in von Willebrand variant and for use of DDAVP. Cryoprecipitate should not be used for a newly diagnosed hemophilia A case, because there are factor concentrates available that have been modified to eliminate the AIDS virus and possibly hepatitis.
Factor VIII concentrate	Quantity of factor VIII units are marked on lyophilized bottle.	25 mL, as per manufacturer's instructions for reconstitution with sterile diluent.	2 yr at 2–8°C storage.	Used for hemophilia A (factor VIII deficiency). Lacks high molecular weight von Willebrand factor. See text for use of DDAVP.
Factor IX concentrate	Contains factors II, VII, IX, and X.	25 mL, as per manufacturer's instructions for reconstitution with sterile diluent.	2 yr at 2–8°C storage.	Most useful for patients with hereditary deficiency of factors II, VII, IX, or X. Sometimes used in patients with high factor VIII antibodies because product contains activated coagulation factors. May cause DIC if severe liver disease present.

Table continued on following page

Table 6–3 □ COMMON BLOOD COMPONENTS AND DERIVATIVES USED IN HEMOTHERAPY *Continued*

Blood Component or Derivative	Characteristics	Approximate Volume	Shelf Life	Indications and Comments
Albumin	5 g/100 mL	250 to 500 mL	3 yr below 30°C.	Most useful for hypovolemic shock or hypoproteinemia.
	25 g/100 mL	50 to 100 mL		Hypertonic (25 g/100 mL) albumin solution rapidly increases intravascular oncotic pressure but draws water from tissues into the intravascular space. Therefore, it is a good idea to monitor arterial and central venous pressure when using this product.
Plasma protein fraction	5 g/100 mL. Contains primarily albumin and some α- and β-globulins.	250 to 500 mL	3 yr below 30°C.	Same as for albumin.
Immune serum globulin	Mostly IgG antibodies, and some IgA and IgM antibodies.	10 mL	3 yr below 30°C.	Treatment or prophylaxis of hypogammaglobulinemia. Prevents and modifies hepatitis A and hepatitis C.
Rh immune globulin	IgG anti-D(Rh$_0$).	1 mL	1½ yr at 2–8°C.	Prevents hemolytic disease of the newborn in Rh-negative women exposed to Rh-positive red cells.

From Henry JB: Clinical Diagnosis and Management by Laboratory Methods, 19th ed. Philadelphia, WB Saunders Co, 1996, p 804.

Risks of Receiving Blood

Risks of not receiving blood in most cases outweigh risks of receiving blood if transfusion is indicated during a surgical procedure or other medical treatment. Some of the well-known risks may include but are not limited to infectious disease and to other adverse effects:

Infectious Disease. Despite careful donor selection and extensive testing of blood products for viruses, the risk of infection cannot be completely eliminated. The reason is that a minimum time must pass before some infectious agents can be detected in donated blood screening tests. The transmission of infectious disease occurs only very rarely and seldom threatens life. The potential risk of contracting AIDS from a blood transfusion has received a great deal of attention. It is important to know that, since 1985, all donated blood in the United States is tested for the AIDS virus, and so the risk is reduced to a negligible level.

Current estimates per unit risk of transmitting infectious agents through blood transfusion are as follows, with recognition that nucleic acid testing (NAT) will reduce this further:

HIV infection is about 1 in 675,000 units transfused

Hepatitis B infection is about 1 in 200,000 units transfused

Hepatitis C infection is about 1 in 103,000 units transfused

HTLV I/II infection is about 1 in 641,000 units transfused

When you consider the risks of transfusion, it may be helpful to recall that many common activities carry far greater risks, e.g., smoking cigarettes, driving a car, or being pregnant.

Other Adverse Effects. Some patients may experience minor changes in the body's immune system after a transfusion, causing mild symptoms, such as fever, chills, or hives, which typically require little or no treatment (1 : 100 to 1 : 150 units transfused). A small number of patients may also react to donated blood by developing antibodies (immune reactions). Other risks include fluid overload, chemical imbalances, breakdown of red blood cells, and possible immunomodulation (alteration in immune system response).

Alternatives to Transfusion

What other choices are there?

- Patient may have other choices to allogeneic (volunteer donor) blood transfusion. Autologous or autogenetic blood transfusion refers to procedures in which patients may serve as their own

Table 6–4 □ BLOOD COMPONENTS AND DERIVATIVES RECOMMENDED FOR VARIOUS CLINICAL CONDITIONS

Clinical Conditions	Preparations Recommended and Comments
Active bleeding	Whole blood or packed red blood cells (RBC), less than 7 days old, if possible, for massive bleeding. Platelets and FFP on occasion for massive bleeding
Anemia: transient	Packed RBC of any acceptable shelf life
Anemia: aplastic	Washed RBC less than 7 days old (to reduce frequency of transfusion and exogenous iron) and/or leukoreduced RBC to decrease HLA exposure
Routine surgery	Whole blood, packed RBC, of any acceptable shelf life
Cardiopulmonary bypass	RBC and crystalloid or colloid solutions. Platelets sometimes necessary when off bypass equipment. Fresh frozen plasma (FFP) needed occasionally
Repeated febrile reactions	Leukoreduced RBC and platelets
Repeated allergic reactions	Washed RBC; washed or plasma reduced platelets
Intrauterine transfusion	CMV-negative group O Rh-negative RBC. Irradiation of RBC should be considered to prevent graft versus host disease if fetus <1200 g or if relative is a directed donor
Exchange transfusion for newborn	CMV-negative whole blood, if available. Packed group O Rh-negative RBC or mother's type less than 7 days old plus 5% albumin. FFP instead of albumin, if coagulation factors are required. Possible irradiation of RBC as for intrauterine transfusion
Immunosuppressed (T-cell)	Leukoreduced, irradiated packed RBC and platelet concentrates and irradiated granulocyte concentrates

Hemodialysis, renal or hepatic failure	Packed RBC
IgA-deficient with anti-IgA requiring transfusion	Washed RBC or blood from IgA-deficient donors
Thrombocytopenia with hemorrhage or impending hemorrhage	Random-donor platelet concentrate. HLA-compatible single-donor apheresed platelets in immunologically refractory patients
Agammaglobulinemia or prevention of hepatitis A, hepatitis B, or hepatitis C	Immune serum globulin, recommended for accidental needle sticks (specific hepatitis A and B immunization is available)
Hemophilia or von Willebrand's disease	DDAVP, if mild to moderate disease: factor VIII concentrate (pasteurized or equivalent safety measures) for severe hemophilia A. DDAVP or Humate-P for von Willebrand's disease (see text for exceptions in certain variants). Cryoprecipitate should be avoided because of risk of infectious complications.
Afibrinogenemia, dysfibrinogenemia, or hypofibrinogenemia	Cryoprecipitate, FFP, no commercial concentrate available
Other coagulopathy	FFP
Shock without hemorrhage	Albumin, other colloids, or crystalloid solutions
Cerebral edema	25% albumin (pulls fluid from tissues into intravascular space) with diuretic therapy
Prevention of Rh sensitization	Rh immune globulin for $RH_0(D)$-negative women to prevent hemolytic disease of the newborn or for inadvertent transfusion of several milliliters of $Rh_0(D)$-positive RBC contained in $Rh_0(D)$-positive blood components such as platelets
Uremia-induced platelet dysfunction	Cryoprecipitate and/or DDAVP
Directed donor—blood relative	Irradiated whole blood or packed RBC

From Henry JB: Clinical Diagnosis and Management by Laboratory Methods, 19th ed. Philadelphia, WB Saunders Co, 1996, p 806.

blood donor. In preoperative autologous donations, the patient's blood may be collected and stored before a scheduled surgery if blood transfusion is likely. In intraoperative and postoperative autologous transfusions, blood lost during surgery is saved and returned to the patient. Directed donations can also be arranged in some cases from a person (usually a friend or relative) whom the patient selects. However, these alternatives also have risks and benefits.

• Some medications may be an alternative to transfusion.

■ BLOOD AND BLOOD COMPONENTS AND DERIVATIVES

Red Blood Cells (RBC)

Red blood cells are transfused to restore oxygen-carrying capacity in patients with symptomatic anemia, anemia and risk or history of cardiovascular or cerebrovascular disease, and actively bleeding patients. A posttransfusion hemoglobin and hematocrit assay should be performed to assess the efficacy of transfusion (a rise of 1 g of hemoglobin or 3% hematocrit after 1 unit).

Indications for Transfusion (Audit Criteria)

Pediatric and Adult Patients
Hemoglobin <7 g/dL or hematocrit <20%
Hemoglobin 7–10 g/dL with signs/symptoms of anemia
Hemoglobin 7–10 g/dL and risk factors or history of cardiovascular or cerebrovascular disease
Hemoglobin >10 g/dL and documented increased O_2 consumption (O_2 extraction ratio >0.50)

Neonates (< 4 months)
Symptomatic anemia. Hemoglobin <8 g/dL or hematocrit <25%
Major surgery. Hemoglobin <10 g/dL or hematocrit <30%
Moderate cardiopulmonary disease. Hemoglobin <10 g/dL or hematocrit <30%
Severe cardiopulmonary disease. Hemoglobin <13 g/dL or hematocrit <40%

RBC Volume

CPDA-1 RBCs. 250 mL/unit (Hct 70–80%)
AS (Adsol) RBCs. 350 mL/unit (Hct 50–60%)

Dose

Adults. 1 unit for each 1-g rise in hemoglobin or 3% rise in hematocrit desired
Neonates and pediatrics. 10 mL/kg of body weight

Administration

Filter. Standard 170 μm (standard blood administration set) (See discussion of universal prestorage leukocyte reduced blood products, p. 67.)

Suggested Rate. Average 2–4 mL/min or about 1–2 hours per unit of ABO and Rh_0-compatible RBC

- A unit of blood must be transfused within 4 hours from release or issue by or from the blood bank. Most patients may be infused over 1–2 hours and average about 90 minutes.
- A slower rate may be required in pediatric patients or adult patients with congestive heart failure, renal failure, or chronic anemia. In these patients, a single unit of red blood cells may need to be split (sterile docking procedure) and transfused as one-fourth unit at a time to meet the 4-hour expiration maximum interval requirement.

Preparation Time

Stat. 60 minutes*
Routine. <4 hours* (average approximately 2 hours)
Routine requests are batched with other work and performed after *stat.* requests are completed. For children less than 1 year of age, fresh units (<7 days of age) are ordered for transfusion. In an emergency, the freshest units in inventory will be used to avoid delay in providing blood.

Specimen

Volume. 7 mL of blood per 3 units ordered (maximum of 21 mL)
Container. Red top, plain
Transport. Room temperature
Other. Red blood cell order form. Specimen and requisition must include patient's full name, medical record number, date, and initials of phlebotomist.

Ordering

The patient must have a current type and crossmatch or a type and screen (T&S) specimen, drawn within the last 72 hours. A signed and completed red blood cell order form, indicating the type of red blood cell product required, total number of units, and the rationale for transfusion, is required at the time blood is or-

---

*Patients with irregular antibodies will require additional time to identify and obtain antigen-negative units. Extra time may also be necessary to obtain special red blood cell products including CMV-seronegative red cells, prestorage leukocyte-reduced red cells, frozen deglycerolized red cells, and washed red cells. See special blood products for additional information (p. 64).

dered and released. The patient should also have a signed, current Consent to Transfuse form in the medical record. Orders for red blood cells are reviewed prospectively at the time of the order and may be referred to the resident or attending pathologist on call or on service for clarification.

Fresh Frozen Plasma (FFP)

Fresh frozen plasma is transfused for the replacement of coagulation factors in patients with a prolonged prothrombin time (PT > 20 seconds, 1.5 times normal, or INR 1.6) and active bleeding or before an invasive procedure. Patients with slightly prolonged PTs (15 to 18 seconds) have sufficient coagulation factor levels for hemostasis. FFP should *not* be prophylactically transfused in a stable, nonbleeding patient with prolonged coagulation studies (as in liver failure), as a volume expander or for nutritional support. A posttransfusion PT/PTT (10 to 20 minutes) should always be performed to assess the efficacy of the transfusion.

Indications (Audit Criteria)

PT >20 seconds and active bleeding or before surgery or an invasive procedure
Active bleeding or trauma, with coagulation studies pending
Documented coagulation factor deficiency with bleeding or before surgery or a procedure
DIC with bleeding or before surgery or a procedure
Post-coronary bypass surgery with microvascular bleeding
Protein S, protein C, or heparin cofactor II deficiency
Emergent reversal of warfarin therapy

Volume

200–250 mL/unit *or*
400–500 mL/unit (FFP collected by apheresis, equivalent to 2 units FFP)

Dose

Adults.   10–15 mL/kg of body weight
Neonates and Pediatrics.   10–15 mL/kg of body weight

Administration

Dispensed as Type-Specific Unless Emergency and Such Unavailable and Then as Type-Compatible
Filter.   Standard 170 μm (standard blood administration set)

Suggested Rate

Before Surgery or Invasive Procedure.   1 unit/hour or 3–4 mL/min, immediately before surgery or procedure.
Bleeding Patient.   As fast a rate as the patient can tolerate.

Preparation Time

15–20 minutes

Specimen

Volume.   7 mL blood if patient's ABO type unknown
Container.   Red top, plain
Transport.   Room temperature
Other.   FFP and cryoprecipitate order form. Specimen and requisition for ABO/Rh type must have patient's full name, medical record number, date, and initials of phlebotomist.

Ordering

The blood bank should be notified at the time the order is placed. Because thawed FFP has a 24-hour shelf life, FFP should be requested only when there are orders to transfuse the product. If the product is not used, the product may be discarded or converted to liquid stored plasma. If the order is canceled, the blood bank should be informed so that the product may be used for another patient. A BCOF must be completed and signed at the time the product is ordered and released. In addition, the patient should have a signed Consent to Transfuse form in the medical record.

All orders for fresh frozen plasma are reviewed prospectively at the time of the initial order. If the results of coagulation studies are normal or pending, the resident will confer with the ordering physician regarding the order.

Thawed Plasma (Liquid Stored Plasma)

Thawed plasma is derived from fresh frozen plasma that has been thawed and stored at 4°C for 1 to 5 days. Thawed plasma contains all the same coagulation factors as FFP except factor V and factor VIII (labile factors), which are reduced. Thawed or liquid stored plasma may be used to treat coagulation-factor deficiencies other than factor VIII. The blood bank can provide liquid stored plasma for emergent reversal of warfarin therapy. Because liquid plasma is immediately available, the blood bank may also provide such plasma for patients in the emergency department or operating room. Liquid stored plasma may be transfused to correct a dilutional coagulopathy while additional FFP is being thawed.

Volume

Same as FFP

Dose

Same as FFP

Administration

Same as FFP

Preparation Time

None

Specimen

Same as FFP

Ordering

Same as FFP

Cryoprecipitate

Cryoprecipitate is prepared from fresh frozen plasma that is allowed to thaw at 4°C and is enriched in fibrinogen, von Willebrand factor, and factor VIII. Each unit of cryoprecipitate contains approximately 250 mg of fibrinogen and 80 to 120 units of factor VIII coagulant activity. Each unit of cryoprecipitate should raise the fibrinogen level approximately 5 mg/dL. If treating a patient with von Willebrand disease or hemophilia A, encourage a Hematology consultation regarding other pharmacologic alternatives.

Indications (Audit Criteria)

Hypofibrinogenemia (fibrinogen <100 mg/dL and bleeding)
Topical fibrin glue (for preparation on site of use)
Von Willebrand disease (consult Hematology)
Hemophilia A (consult Hematology)
Uremia with bleeding (Table 6–5), unresponsive to desmopressin
   (DDAVP) and dialysis
(Hematology and Nephrology consultation suggested)

Table 6–5 □ OPTIONS FOR PATIENTS WITH UREMIA
AND BLEEDING*

Treatment	Purpose
1. Dialysis	Improve platelet function
2. Maintain hematocrit >24%	Bleeding time increases when Hct <24%
3. Maintain platelets >70,000/μL	Augment level of partially functional platelets
4. Administer conjugated estrogen 0.6 mg/kg iv qd × 5d	Effective in 6 hours; maximal correction in 5 days; lasts 14 days
5. Administer desmopressin (DDAVP) 0.3 μg/kg iv q12–24 hr × 2	Releases endothelial von Willebrand factor; effective in 30–60 minutes May not be effective with continued dosing

*Check PT/PTT and give FFP if indicated.   > = Greater than
 Check for anatomic defect as source of bleeding.   < = Less than

Volume

10–15 mL/unit

Dose

Hypofibrinogenemia (fibrinogen <100 mg/dL)
Adults.   8–10 units (or 1 unit per 7 kg of body weight)
Neonates and Pediatrics.   1 unit per 5–7 kg of body weight
Topical Fibrin Glue.   2 units of thawed cryoprecipitate for on site preparation and use.
Von Willebrand Disease, Hemophilia A, or Uremic Bleeding.
May require Hematology consultation

Administration

Filter.   Standard 170 μm (standard blood administration set)
Rate.   1–4 mL/min
Preparation Time.   20 minutes

Specimen

Volume.   7 mL blood if patient's ABO type unknown
Container.   Red top, plain
Transport.   Room temperature
Other.   FFP and cryoprecipitate order form. Specimen and requisition for ABO type must have patient's full name, medical record number, date, and initials of phlebotomist.

Ordering

The blood bank should be notified when one is ordering cryoprecipitate. Cryoprecipitate has a 4-hour shelf life after thawing and pooling and should be requested with orders only when it is to be transfused. If not used, the thawed product may be discarded. A BCOF must be signed and completed at the time the order is placed and released. The patient should also have a current, signed Consent to Transfuse form in the medical record. All initial orders for cryoprecipitate are reviewed by the resident or pathologist on call.

Platelets

Platelet concentrates may be required to treat or prevent bleeding in thrombocytopenic patients. Platelet concentrates are available as random donor platelets pooled, "whole blood-derived" platelet concentrates, or single-donor apheresis platelet concentrates. Pooled, whole blood-derived platelet concentrates are usually provided in response to routine orders. Except for bone marrow and peripheral blood-progenitor cell transplant and oncology patients, all initial requests for single-donor apheresis platelet concentrates must be approved by the resident or pathologist on call.

A 10-minute to 1-hour posttransfusion platelet count *must* be performed after *each* platelet transfusion to measure the efficacy of transfusion. This step is particularly important in multitransfused patients or multiparous females who may develop immune refractoriness to platelets. If a patient is not responding clinically to platelets infusions (a posttransfusion increment <10,000), an evaluation for HLA or crossmatched platelets (see p. 69) should be considered. An appropriate blood specimen should also be sent to the HLA laboratory to test for the presence of lymphocytotoxic antibodies (anti-HLA) or percent reactive antibody (PRA) assay with HLA typing if not available.

A corrected count increment (CCI) calculation for assessment of effectiveness of platelet transfusions is as follows:

$$CCI = \frac{PI \times BSA}{n}$$

PI = Platelet increment

BSA = Body surface area (square meters)

n = Number of platelets transfused ($\times 10^{11}$)

CCI should approximate 7500 at 1 hour

Indications (Audit Criteria)

Platelet count <10,000/μL

Platelet count 10,000–20,000/μL and additional risk factors for bleeding or for an outpatient

Platelet count <50,000/μL and currently bleeding, before surgery or invasive procedure

Platelet count <100,000/μL on ECMO, or scheduled for neurosurgery, eye or airway surgery

Platelet function defect and bleeding (i.e., inherited platelet defect, recent administration of monoclonal anti-IIb/IIIa) or salicylate daily therapy in a patient going to surgery

Volume

Whole Blood Derived.   50 mL/unit (7.5 $\times 10^{10}$ platelets total)
Apheresis.   300–500 mL/unit (3.0–5.0 $\times 10^{11}$ platelets)

Dose

Adults.

5–6 units of pooled platelet concentrate (~4.0 $\times 10^{11}$ platelets per 250–300 mL)

1 unit of apheresis platelet concentrate (~4.0 $\times 10^{11}$ platelets per 350 mL)

Pediatrics.   10 mL/kg of body weight
Neonates.   10 mL/kg of body weight

Administration

Filter. Standard 170 μm (standard blood administration set)
(For leukocyte-reduced platelets, an appropriate leukocyte-reduction filter may be necessary. See p. 67.)

Suggested Rate

2–4 mL/min or approximately 1 unit/hour

Preparation Time

20 minutes (pooled platelet concentrate)

Specimen

Volume. 7 mL blood if patient ABO/Rh type unknown
Container. Red top, plain
Transport. Room temp
Other. Platelet Order Form. Specimen and requisition sent for ABO/Rh type. Specimen and requisition must have patient's full name, medical record number, date, and initials of phlebotomist.

Ordering

The blood bank should be called when one is ordering platelet products. A platelet order form must be signed and completed at the time platelets are ordered and released. The patient should also have a current, signed Consent to Transfuse form in the medical record. All orders for platelets are reviewed at the time of the order and may be referred to the resident and ordering physician for clarification.

Because platelets have a brief storage interval or shelf life (5 days), platelets should be ordered at the time when a decision to transfuse has been made by the responsible physician. A small inventory of platelets is kept in stock. Therefore it is not necessary or appropriate to request platelets "on call." Once pooled, platelets have a shelf life of 4 hours. If an order is canceled, the blood bank should be notified promptly so that the product can be used for another patient.

Albumin (Derivative)

Albumin is frequently used to correct and maintain a sufficient intravascular volume and tissue perfusion as a volume expander in patients. Albumin is available as a 5% and 25% solution. 5% albumin solution is osmotically and oncotically equivalent to plasma. A 25% albumin solution is hypertonic and hyperosmotic relative to blood and must be diluted accordingly with normal saline (NS) before transfusion.

Indications

Hypovolemia or hypotension unresponsive to 20–50 mL/kg of crystalloid

Burn patient >24 hours

Paracentesis >4 liters of ascitic fluid

Nephrotic syndrome (with use of a diuretic)

Therapeutic plasma exchange

Intravascular volume depletion with interstitial fluid excess, i.e., edema

Volume

5% Albumin.   250 mL (12.5 g of protein total)
25% Albumin.   50 mL (12.5 g of protein total)

Collection Instructions

Albumin order form

Specimen

None

Comments

Patients with hypovolemia or hypotension should initially be resuscitated with crystalloid solutions (NS, lactated Ringer's) or Hespan (6% hetastarch in 500 mL of NS, up to 20 mL/kg/24 hours). NOTE: Do not use Hespan in patients with underlying bleeding disorders.

Before transfusion, 25% albumin should be diluted with an isotonic solution such as normal saline. Intravascular hemolysis has been reported after transfusion of albumin diluted with water.

■ SPECIAL BLOOD PRODUCTS

Autologous Red Blood Cells

Patients undergoing elective surgery may predeposit autologous blood before surgery. Patients suitable for autologous donation are those patients undergoing procedures in which blood transfusion is likely, i.e., *type and crossmatch > 2 units.* Autologous blood should *not* be collected in patients undergoing procedures requiring only a T&S (Table 6–2).

Indications

Type and crossmatch ≥2 units

Estimated surgical blood loss >1000 mL or 10% total blood volume

Patients with multiple red blood cell alloantibodies

Patients with alloantibodies to high incidence of antigens

Women who have had multiple pregnancies

Collection Instructions and Ordering

An order for autologous blood collection must be initiated by the requesting physician.

Patient Requirements

12–70 years of age
Hematocrit >33%
Absence of infection
More than 72 hours after dental procedure or other surgical manipulation (e.g., cystoscopy)
Absence of a significant underlying medical condition predisposing to a cardiovascular event or vasovagal reaction after removal of 500 mL of blood.
Adequate venous access (blood cannot be drawn from central lines or catheters)
Patients should call to schedule appointments.

Turnaround

One unit a week, up to 5 working days before surgery.

Comments

Patients should start oral ferrous sulfate supplementation before donation and surgery. Recommended adult dose is 300 mg po tid.

Directed-Donor Red Blood Cells

Patients in whom autologous donation is not possible because of illness, age, or low hematocrit may have blood donated for them by select individuals. Directed donors must be ABO/Rh and cross-match compatible with the patient. In addition, directed donors must meet the same eligibility requirements for whole blood donation as volunteer blood donors. Because of the time required to schedule, collect, and test donor units, directed-donor red blood cells are not available in emergency situations.

Potential donors *must* have proof of their ABO/Rh type at the time of initial donation. Directed-donor units may be used only by the patient for whom it was donated. Directed-donor red cell units must be crossmatched before transfusion. Unused units will be discarded.

Collection Instructions and Ordering

An order for directed-donor blood collection must be initiated by the requesting physician. The appropriate completed forms and a patient specimen for a T&S must be submitted. If the potential donor or donors do not have documentation of their ABO/Rh type, a specimen for a T&S on the donor should also be sent.

Donor Requirements

Same as volunteer blood donors

Documented proof of ABO/Rh type at initial donation
Potential donors should call donor or hemotherapy center to schedule appointments.

Turnaround Time

5 working days

Specimen

Volume.   7 mL of blood
Container.   Red top, plain
Transport.   Room temperature
Other.   Completed form by requesting physician

Specimens for ABO/Rh typing must have patient's full name, medical record number, date, and initials of phlebotomist.

Comments

A directed donor may donate only 1 unit of whole blood each 56 days. A patient requiring more then 1 unit of blood will require multiple donors to fulfill his or her transfusion requirements.

Cytomegalovirus (CMV)-seronegative and CMV-safe Red Blood Cells and Platelets

CMV-seronegative blood products may be indicated in certain patients. CMV-seronegative patients at risk for transfusion-associated CMV infection may require transfusion with CMV-seronegative blood products. Alternatively, such patients may be transfused with CMV random, leukocyte-reduced red blood cells and platelets. The latter have been shown to be "CMV safe" and equivalent to CMV seronegative. Products capable of transmitting CMV are red blood cells and platelets; FFP and cryoprecipitate do not contain viable lymphocytes and thus are unable to transmit CMV. Overall, the risk of transfusion-associated CMV infection from a (nonleukocyte-reduced) CMV-seropositive red cell or platelet product is $<0.03\%$ per unit.

Indications for CMV Seronegative Products

Pregnant and CMV seronegative
Intrauterine transfusions
Neonates <4 months of age and <1300 g from CMV-seronegative mothers
CMV-seronegative allogeneic bone marrow transplant candidates

CMV-seronegative allogeneic bone marrow transplant recipient transplanted with bone marrow from a CMV-seronegative donor

Other (pathology resident approval required)

Patients Receiving CMV Safe (Leukocyte Reduced)

CMV-seronegative autogeneic bone marrow (BM) and peripheral blood (PB) progenitor cell (PC) transplant recipients

CMV-seropositive allogeneic BM and PB PC candidates

CMV-seronegative allogeneic BM and PB, PC transplant recipients transplanted with BM from a CMV-positive donor

CMV-seronegative renal transplant recipient or candidate

CMV-seronegative oncology patients

Other (pathology resident approval required)

Preparation Time

Dependent on product availability

Specimens

Same as for platelets or red cells. If CMV status of patient is unknown, a CMV serology assay must be ordered.

Ordering

If CMV-seronegative products are not available for patients requiring CMV-seronegative products, the resident or pathologist on call will contact the ordering physician regarding the urgency of the transfusion and other options. All initial orders for CMV-seronegative products are reviewed by the resident on call.

Leukocyte-reduced Blood Products

Leukocyte-reduced red blood cells and platelets are provided for transplant patients or candidates or patients requiring long-term transfusion support to prevent alloimmunization. Leukocyte-reduced red cells have also been shown to prevent cytomegalovirus infections and are considered "CMV safe." Prestorage leukocyte reduction has also been shown to reduce the incidence of febrile transfusion reactions by preventing the accumulation of leukocyte-derived inflammatory cytokines.

Leukocytes may be removed at the time of transfusion by use of commercial leukocyte-reduction filters (bedside leukofiltration) or may be leukocyte reduced at the time of collection (prestorage leukocyte reduced).* Other than renal and bone marrow transplant candidates or recipients, all initial requests for prestorage leukocyte-reduced* red blood cells and platelets will be reviewed by the resident on call until universal prestorage leukocyte reduction of blood products is available.

---

*Universal prestorage leukocyte reduction for RBC and platelets is evolving currently in the USA.

Indications for Leukocyte-reduced Blood Products (Audit Criteria)

Bone marrow or peripheral blood progenitor cell (PC) transplant candidate or recipient

Renal transplant candidate or recipient

Intrauterine transfusion

Solid organ transplant recipient

Hematologic malignancy

Hemoglobinopathy patients requiring long-term transfusion support

Patients with a history of repeated, severe transfusion reactions despite appropriate premedication (pathology resident approval required)*

Other (pathology resident approval required)

Prestorage leukocyte-reduced

Preparation Time

Bedside leukofiltration, none

Prestorage leukocyte-reduced, dependent on product availability

Ordering

If prestorage leukocyte-reduced products are needed, contact the blood bank at the time the order is initiated. Depending on local availability, it may take several hours to obtain a prestorage leukocyte-reduced product. If there will be a significant delay in filling the order, the resident or pathologist on call will contact the ordering physician regarding the urgency of the transfusion and other options. All initial orders for leukocyte-reduced blood products are reviewed by the resident on call.

Irradiated Red Blood Cells and Platelets

Certain patients may require irradiated blood products to prevent transfusion-associated graft-versus-host disease (GVHD, see p. 96). Products that require irradiation include red blood cells and platelets; FFP and cryoprecipitate do not contain viable lymphocytes and therefore do not require irradiation.

Indications (audit criteria)

Bone marrow or peripheral blood progenitor cell (PC) transplant candidates or recipients

Hematologic malignancy

Congenital immunodeficiency

---

*Universal prestorage leukocyte reduction for RBC and platelets is evolving currently in the USA.

Aplastic anemia

Intrauterine transfusions

Neonates <1300 g and <4 months of age

HLA-matched platelets

Solid organ malignancy undergoing intense, multiagent chemotherapy

Directed-donor blood products from relatives

Other (pathology resident approval required)

NOTE: In general, solid organ transplant recipients and patients
with AIDS do **not** require irradiated blood products.

Preparation Time

15 minutes

Ordering

The blood bank should be notified when an order for irradiated
products is initiated. All initial orders for irradiated products will
be reviewed by the resident. Products are irradiated immediately
before use. *Contact the blood bank again approximately 15 minutes before the time the product is to be picked up for transfusion.*

HLA-matched Platelets

Some patients may fail to respond appropriately to platelet
transfusion. On average, a pool of 6 whole blood-derived platelet
concentrates or a single apheresis platelet concentrate should result in a 30,000 to 60,000 rise in the platelet count by 1 hour after
transfusion. A patient who fails to undergo an increment by 10,000
should be evaluated for platelet refractoriness. Refractoriness may
be attributable to nonimmune factors (fever, sepsis, disseminated
intravascular coagulation [DIC], antilymphocytic globulin [ALG]
administration) or may reflect immune refractoriness because of
anti-HLA or specific platelet antibodies. Patients who are at particular risk for immune platelet refractoriness caused by HLA antibodies are multiparous females and multitransfused patients. All
orders for HLA-matched platelets must be referred to the resident
or pathologist on call.

Criteria for HLA-matched Platelets

Bone marrow or peripheral blood progenitor cell (PC) transplant
candidate or recipient with a known anti-HLA (antibody).

or

The absence of nonimmune causes for refractoriness *and* a corrected count increment (CCI) <7000 in three consecutive platelet
transfusions or a CCI <7000 in the majority of five platelet transfusions.

Preparation Time (initial order)

1–48 hours depending on product availability

Specimen Requirements (initial order)

7 mL, plain red tube (no gel) for HLA antibody screen and 20 mL, two green (sodium heparin) plus one purple (Versene) tube for complete HLA typing.

Ordering

HLA-matched platelets require communication with the Transfusion Medicine resident (8:00–5:00 weekdays) or Clinical Pathology resident on call (evenings and weekends). The resident and attending will review the patient's transfusion record, clinical course, and history to determine whether HLA-matched platelets are appropriate in the patient. Refractoriness must be documented by a 1-hour posttransfusion platelet count and a posttransfusion corrected count increment (CCI) less than 7000.

To receive HLA-matched platelets, the patient must have an HLA type on file. A screen for HLA antibodies should also be sent on all initial requests for HLA-matched platelets. If an HLA type is not known, a specimen should be sent for typing to the HLA laboratory. If an HLA type cannot be performed for technical reasons (blast crises, leukopenia), antigen-negative products or cross-matched platelets may be provided as determined by the Transfusion Medicine fellow or attending and ordering physician.

Solvent-Detergent-treated Plasma

Solvent-detergent-treated plasma (SD plasma) is a modified pooled plasma product approved by the FDA. Pooled plasma from 2500 donors is treated with a solvent-detergent process to inactivate lipid-enveloped viruses such as HIV, HCV, and HBV. SD plasma contains factor levels equivalent to FFP except that SD plasma is deficient in high-molecular-weight von Willebrand factor multimers. SD plasma does not inactivate nonenveloped viruses such as hepatitis A or human parvovirus B19.

Our hospital transfusion subcommittee has recommended prior approval by the Transfusion Medicine physician or Hematology for all initial requests for SD plasma. The latter reflects the pooled nature of SD plasma and potential infection risk by nonenveloped viruses when compared to the low theoretical risk of HIV, HCV, and HBV transmission from tested, single-donor non-SD treated FFP. SD plasma may be appropriate in patients requiring intense or long-term support with FFP only. For patients requiring plasma and either red blood cell or platelet transfusion support, SD plasma may not be appropriate (e.g., for a surgical patient). SD plasma may not be appropriate in immunosuppressed, pregnant patients, or patients with chronic hemolytic states attributable to the theoretical transmission of parvovirus B19. Parvovirus B19 has been associated with aplastic cases, pure red blood cell aplasia, hydrops fetalis, and pancytopenia.

■ ROLE OF RESIDENT ON CALL

Calls over the course of a year include:

Evaluation of Requests for Blood Products

Red blood cells
Fresh frozen plasma
Cryoprecipitate
Platelets

Transfusion Reaction and Report

Hemolytic transfusion reaction
Febrile transfusion reaction
Allergic transfusion reaction
Hypervolemia or circulatory overload

Evaluation of Requests for Special Blood Products

Leukocyte-reduced blood products
Irradiated blood products
IgA-deficient blood products
CMV-negative blood products

Massive Transfusion

T&S versus Type & Crossmatch

Incompatible Crossmatch

Alloantibody Identification and Report

Role of resident on call is subsequently considered in light of the above. The response to call will be most effective and efficient with concurrent review of Policies and Procedure (p. 32), Blood and Blood Components and Derivatives (p. 56), Special Blood Products (p. 64), and five expanded major topics: Emergency Transfusion (p. 77), Massive Transfusion (p. 81), Incompatible Crossmatch (p. 83), Transfusion Reactions (pp. 44 and 88), and Rh Immune Globulin (RhIG) (p. 97).

Review Requests

- Fresh frozen plasma: more than 4 units per patient or any volume in a patient with normal coagulation studies.
- Platelets: single donor units, HLA-matched apheresis products. All platelet requests, especially those exceeding 6 random-donor pooled units should be reviewed to determine if appropriate.
- Leukocyte-reduced packed red cells, washed red cells, frozen red cells, requests for irradiated blood.
- Clarification and confirmation of patient's needs including laboratory monitors and clinical condition often suffice.

Contact ordering physician if *blood component order form (BCOF)* does not have an appropriate indication and rationale noted. Consult with attending pathologist if necessary in unusual circumstances. Record changes in orders and rationale for unusual orders on BCOF (see Figs. 6–3 to 6–6). If an order is not changed and seems inappropriate, bring information to attention for review by Blood Utilization Review Committee. Follow up cases for whom orders were canceled. Note any adverse outcomes that may have resulted from use of the guidelines (see Table 6–2).

Calls pertaining to what appear to be *transfusion reactions* are an emergency. These require a thorough, prompt transfusion-reaction workup (see discussion of transfusion reactions, pp. 44 and 88, and Fig. 6–7).

Follow up transfusion reactions by ascertaining present status of patient, necessary emergency therapy, if any, desired follow-up laboratory assessment, and future blood requirements from clinicians with a prompt verbal preliminary report back to clinicians. Any hemolytic transfusion reaction requires your presence at the bedside immediately and to telephone promptly the attending pathologist. Present written report to attending pathologist within 24 hours including weekends (Fig. 6–8) (see p. 44).

Check the *blood bank inventory* and be aware of any *blood shortages* (especially O-negative RBC and group AB FFP), keeping in mind potential and actual demands (see Tables 6–1 to 6–4).

Be aware of antibody workups in progress and communicate antibody or crossmatch problems (p. 83) to the appropriate clinician (Fig. 6–9). Review blood orders for next-day surgery and compare operating room schedule orders with *Guidelines for Ordering Blood for Elective Surgery* (see Table 6–2). Observe deviations greater than guidelines and seek clarification and confirmation, i.e., predisposing condition; also suggest preferred use of T&S to type and crossmatch (specified number of units) with rapid TAT assured.

Depending on total blood products utilized over a defined time frame, a minimal inventory of each product is maintained. Resident on call should at all times be aware of this inventory including *sudden and substantial product depletions,* i.e., in patients with trauma or perioperative bleeding, coagulopathies, and acquired disorders of hemostasis (see Chapter 9). Other clinical challenges beyond balancing blood product inventory with *sudden and often unexpected patient needs for blood products* are immunosuppressed (or immunosuppression-anticipated) patients requiring leukocyte-reduced, irradiated, and CMV-negative blood products.

Immunized or sensitized patients with autoantibodies, irregular antibodies, HLA or cytotoxic antibodies, and incompatible crossmatch needing resolution can often involve the resident on call in special coordination and communication with clinical colleagues

UNIVERSITY HOSPITAL
BLOOD BANK/TRANSFUSION MEDICINE
TRANSFUSION REACTION EVALUATION

All information must be completed to facilitate prompt laboratory evaluation

Date _7/10/99_   Time Blood Bank notified of reaction _1530_   (ext. 46700)
Blood unit number _OIGN29139_   Component transfused: ☐ Red cells ☐ Platelets ☐ Plasma ☐ Cryoprecipitate
Time transfusion initiated _1330_   Time terminated _1520_   Amount of product transfused _264_ mL

BEDSIDE CLERICAL CHECK: Did patient wristband information match that on the transfusion tag? ☑ Yes ☐ No

Vital signs: Blood pressure   Before transfusion _112/42_   At time transfusion was terminated _140/64_
              Body temperature Before transfusion _372_   At time transfusion was terminated _361_
              Pulse   Before transfusion _80_   At time transfusion was terminated _80_

Symptoms/Signs Present: (Check all that apply)
☑ Chills   ☐ Fever   ☐ Chest pain ☐ Shortness of breath ☐ Back pain ☐ Hypotension ☐ Hemoglobinuria
☐ Nausea ☐ Flushing ☐ Hives/Rash ☐ Wheezing   ☑ Headache ☐ Hypertension ☐ Tachycardia

Other Clinical Findings and Assessment:

_____ Nurse signature

nail beds - blue

color-skin - pale

_____ MD

INITIAL EVALUATION

Clerical check performed: All information on specimens, requisitions, and donor units correct? ☑ Yes ☐ No
Hemolysis Check: Free Hgb in post-trans. serum _Neg_   Free hgb in post-trans. urine _Neg_
Free hgb in pre-trans. serum _Neg_

	Anti-A	Anti-B	A1 Cells	B Cells	Anti-D	D Control	AHG	Anti-IgG	Anti-C3	Pos. Cont.	Interpretation
	ABO Grouping				Rh Typing		Recipient DAT				
Recipient's pre-transfusion specimen	0	0	++++	++++	+++	0				++	OPos, Neg DA
Recipient's post-transfusion specimen	0	0	++++	++++	+++	0				++	OPos, Neg DA
Unit no. _OIGN 29139_ (segment/aliquot)	0	0			+++						OPos,

☐ No further work indicated

	SI	SII	SI	SII	Pos. Cont.	I.S.	37 C	AHG	Pos. Cont.	Interpretation
	Screening for Irregular Antibodies 37 C / AHG					Crossmatch with Bag Segment or Aliquot				
Recipient's pre-transfusion specimen						0	0	0	++	Comp
Recipient's post-transfusion specimen						0	0	0	++	Comp

Megan McElligott Blood Bank Technologist

OTHER EXAMINATIONS/MEASUREMENTS:
Gram stain on blood bag: Culture on residual:

CLINICAL IMPRESSION & FOLLOW-UP: (Please see reverse)   C24.00 - Rev 11/97

Figure 6–8A ☐ Example of a completed transfusion reaction evaluation form (obverse side).

Illustration continued on following page

UNIVERSITY HOSPITAL
BLOOD BANK/TRANSFUSION MEDICINE
TRANSFUSION REACTION EVALUATION

CLINICAL IMPRESSION AND FOLLOW-UP

CLINICAL EVALUATION: The patient is a 69 year old white female (G3P3) who was transferred to University Hospital on 7/7/99. She had resection arthroplasty of left hip with insertion of antibiotic impregnated cement spacer on 6/23/99 for an infected hip prosthesis. Subsequently the patient was transferred to the rehabilitation unit at University Hospital. Her medical history is significant for coronary artery disease, two myocardial infarctions in the past, hypertension, diabetes mellitus type II, frequent urinary tract infections and chronic anemia. Patient has had cholecystectomy, bowel resection for diverticulosis, and left THA in the past. She received autologous transfusion of packed red cells (one unit) during the left total hip arthroplasty and one more unit of regular packed red cells from a separate donor in the postoperative period in April 1999. She developed a non hemolytic febrile transfusion reaction during the second transfusion. Additionally the patient was transfused with one unit of prestorage leukoreduced packed red cells in June 1999 at the time of the recent left hip resection arthroplasty. Patient has no history of anti-HLA antibodies, however she has an anti-Kell alloantibody.

   On 7/10/99, the patient was transfused with (OIGN29139) one unit of packed red cells as she had a hematocrit of 25%. The patient was premedicated with Benadryl and Tylenol prior to transfusion. After transfusion of 264 mL the patient complained of chills. On examination cyanosis was evident in her nail beds and the skin was pale. The patient's vital signs pre-transfusion were BP: 112/42, Pulse: 80, Temperature: 37.2° Celsius. Post-transfusion vital signs were BP: 140/64, Pulse: 80, Temperature: 36.1° Celsius. However thirty minutes after the transfusion was stopped the patient's temperature rose to 37.5 from 36.1° Celsius. Her oxygen saturation was 97%.

Laboratory Evaluation: The patient typed as O, Rh positive on repeat testing of the pre- and post-transfusion samples. The donor unit was O, Rh positive and was ABO compatible with the donor. Additionally the unit was negative for the Kell antigen. There were no clerical errors. Pre- and post-transfusion direct antiglobulin tests were negative. A post-transfusion serum sample showed no visible hemolysis. Post-transfusion urine sample was negative for hemoglobinuria.

Impression: Though there was an initial drop in the patient's body temperature, there was a subsequent elevation. This finding together with patient's signs and symptoms are most suggestive of a febrile, nonhemolytic, transfusion reaction.

Febrile reactions are commonly associated with the transfusion of white cell-derived cytokines which accumulate during blood storage. Febrile reactions may also result from anti-platelet or anti-leukocyte antibodies in the recipient which react with transfused donor cells. Premedication with Tylenol is suggested prior to transfusion. In some patients, premedication with diphenhydramine (Benadryl), demerol, or hydrocortisone may be necessary.

Additionally, as this patient has history of prior febrile transfusion reactions, we recommend use of leukoreduced packed red cells in the future.

_____ MD
Pathology Resident

_____ MD
Blood Bank/Transfusion Medicine Attending*

*I have reviewed the available clinical history and laboratory results, reviewed the interpretation of the resident, made editorial changes where appropriate and completed the final diagnosis.

C24.00 - Rev 11/97

Figure 6–8B □ Example of a completed transfusion reaction evaluation form (reverse side).

STATE UNIVERSITY OF NEW YORK
Health Science Center at Syracuse

CLINICAL PATHOLOGY - SPECIAL

DATE: August 25,1999

IMMUNOHEMATOLOGY REPORT

BLOOD TYPE: A, Rho(D) positive, Kell negative

ANTIBODY IDENTIFIED: Anti-Kell

CLINICAL SIGNIFICANCE: Causes Transfusion Reactions: yes

DIFFICULTY IN FINDING COMPATIBLE BLOOD:

☑ No Problem   ☐ May Take Some Time   ☐ Difficult

COMMENTS: This is a 61 year old male with coronary artery disease, status post coronary artery bypass grafting surgery in 1988, admitted at this time with unstable angina requiring cardiac catheterization and angioplasty. His medical history also includes rheumatoid arthritis, type II diabetes mellitus, hypertension, hemorrhoids, and hyperlipidemia. His transfusion history is not documented in the medical record.

At this time, anti-Kell is detected in the patient's serum. The patient's serum reacted with one of two screening cells and 3/12 panel cells in the antiglobulin phase. An autocontrol was negative. Anti-Kell was identified and all other antibodies were excluded.

Anti-Kell is usually an IgG antibody which results from previous sensitization via transfusion. Anti-Kell is associated with hemolytic transfusion reactions.

If red cell transfusion is necessary, Kell-negative donor units will be provided. Approximately 91% ot type-specific donors will be compatible and a full crossmatch will be necessary before blood can be transfused. Extra time will be necessary to find compatible units.

Sharad C. Mathur, M.D.
Pathology Resident

John Bernard Henry, M.D.
Attending Clinical Pathologist*

☑ Antibody Consult
   Comprehensive

☑ Billing entered into
   lab computer by _LY_

*I have reviewed the available clinical history, the laboratory results, and the interpretation of the resident/fellow, made editorial changes where appropriate, and I confirm the final interpretation and recommended hemotherapy.

Figure 6–9 □ Immunohematology report: antibody against Kell blood group antigen.

and blood bank technologists (see discussion of incompatible crossmatch, p. 83).

Massive transfusion (p. 88) cases (actual or potential) are emergencies that warrant prompt follow-up study with evaluation and assessment including a visit to the operating room or the Emergency Medicine department. Interaction and communication with clinicians then permits anticipation of specific blood component needs, i.e., number and variety of units and over what period of time (Tables 6–6 and 6–7). Communication of this information to blood bank technologists and coordinating blood bank

Table 6–6 □ ETIOLOGY OF MASSIVE TRANSFUSION

Hypovolemic/hemorrhagic shock from excessive blood loss:
- Gastrointestinal (GI) hemorrhage
  Esophageal-gastric varices bleeding
  Peptic ulcer bleeding
- Ruptured aortic aneurysm
- Complex/complicated surgery
  Redo coronary artery bypass
  Prosthetic/autograft valve(s) replacement
- Trauma
  Motor vehicular accidents (MVA)
  Multiple penetrating wounds
  ○ Knife/bullets
- Transplantation of liver

product support with clinicians and technical staff become a high priority.

Neonatal hemotherapy often has a combination of requirements. Neonatal period extends to the fourth month of life. Blood volume (BV) at full term is about 85 mL/kg, whereas premature babies are less than 1200 g and BV can exceed 100 mL/kg. Hence, special needs for neonatal intensive care units, pediatric surgery, and pediatric (ICU) patients for hemotherapy include CPD-A1 anticoagulated red blood cells less than 7 days old or as whole blood and often and preferably O negative but drawn into four discrete units; these integrally attached packs employing sterile docking technology and are dispensed for infusion in aliquots accordingly. Irradiation and CMV-negative, hemoglobin S-negative, and leukocyte-reduced packed red cells are most appropriate with low birth weight

Table 6–7 □ POTENTIAL COMPLICATIONS OF MASSIVE TRANSFUSION

- Hypothermia secondary to infusion of cold fluids rapidly and loss of thermal regulation
- Electrolyte imbalance:
  Hypokalemia often with depressed serum magnesium
  Hyperkalemia with renal failure and in neonates
  Hypocalcemia caused by excess citrate reflected most sensitively in plasma-ionized calcium measurements if not symptoms
- Cardiac arrythmias secondary to electrolyte imbalance and acidemia
- Coagulation and hemostasis abnormalities:
  Dilutional
  Consumption
  Dysfunctional platelets
- Hypervolemia/circulatory overload

and prematurity. RBC products collected from a blood donor relative also should be irradiated.

Rh immune globulin (RhIG) calls are most often for an unimmunized Rh_0 (D)-negative pregnant woman usually at 28 to 30 weeks (may be up to 38 weeks) of gestation and again at term or delivery within 72 hours of giving birth to an Rh_0 (D)-positive infant. It is **not administered** if she has preexisting antibody as anti-Rh_0 (D) in her serum or her newborn baby is Rh_0 (D) negative. Hence mother's blood must be ABO and Rh_0 (D) typed and screened for preexisting anti-Rh_0 (D). RhIG is usually dispensed by the pharmacy in a 1-mL vial as a full dose sufficient to counteract the immunizing effect of 15 mL of Rh_0 (D)-positive red blood cells. RhIG is also indicated after abortion, antepartum hemorrhage, amniocentesis, chorionic villus sampling, ectopic pregnancies, and fetal death. Further use of RhIG and its use as an alternative to intravenous immunoglobulin (IVIgG) is considered subsequently (p. 97).

Immunized patients with autoantibodies may require ABO or group O Rh_0-matched red blood cell products with least-incompatible crossmatch or biologic *in vivo* crossmatch (50-mL infusion and concurrent patient monitoring and assessment). Likewise, patients with irregular antibodies require appropriate antigen-negative products and completed form (Figs. 6–9 to 6–11 and see the discussion of incompatible crossmatch, p. 83).

ABO grouping discrepancies, called to your attention, should always first be repeated to rule out any clerical or technical error. When results are then unchanged, problems with either the patient's serum or patient's cells need to be reviewed (Table 6–8). In an emergency and if any discrepancy cannot be resolved in a timely manner, group O packed red blood cells, AB fresh frozen plasma, or both may be given.

■ EMERGENCY TRANSFUSION

Uncrossmatched and ABO Type-specific Units

Emergencies often prompt release of uncrossmatched group O, Rh_0 (D)-negative units though ABO- and Rh_0-compatible units are always preferable if time permits. Regular compatibility testing or at least a T&S should then be done as quickly as possible to provide any additional units crossmatched. Notify clinician if any incompatibility is detected in such follow-up crossmatches after such emergency releases or infusions with delineation of incompatibility. A transfusion-reaction workup should be performed when an alloantibody is identified in patient transfused *stat.* with group O, Rh_0 (D)-negative units if the unit was incompatible on subsequent testing.

STATE UNIVERSITY OF NEW YORK
Health Science Center at Syracuse

CLINICAL PATHOLOGY - SPECIAL

DATE: August 25, 1999

IMMUNOHEMATOLOGY REPORT

BLOOD TYPE: O, Rho(D) positive, M positive, Le^a negative, Le^b positive, P$_1$ negative

ANTIBODY IDENTIFIED: Non-specific cold agglutinin

CLINICAL SIGNIFICANCE: Causes Transfusion Reactions: yes

DIFFICULTY IN FINDING COMPATIBLE BLOOD:

☑ No Problem   ☐ May Take Some Time   ☐ Difficult

COMMENTS: This patient is a 74 year old male with coronary artery disease and mitral valve insufficiency, currently being evaluated for surgery on 8/26/99. No other clinical history could be obtained.
    This patient has a cold agglutinin which is reactive with 2/2 screening cells and 2/11 panel cells at room temperature and is weakly reactive with one screening cell in the antiglobulin phase of testing. A thermal amplitude study showed agglutination at 26°C. All 37°C reactive alloantibodies have been ruled out. An autocontrol was negative. Should this patient require transfusion, blood compatible by prewarming technique will be provided.

Sharad C. Mathur, M.D.
Sharad C. Mathur, M.D.
Pathology Resident

John Bernard Henry, M.D.
John Bernard Henry, M.D.
Attending Clinical Pathologist*

☑ Antibody Consult
  Comprehensive

☑ Billing entered into
  lab computer by _LY_

*I have reviewed the available clinical history, the laboratory results, and the interpretation of the resident/fellow, made editorial changes where appropriate, and I confirm the final interpretation and recommended hemotherapy.

Figure 6–10 □ Immunohematology report: cold agglutinin.

The emergency-transfusion response should therefore initially consist in providing or releasing uncrossmatched ABO/Rh type-specific RBC unit or units if one assumes that there is sufficient time. Depending on technical staffing, time of day, and concurrent demands, T&S may require up to an hour (or usually 20 minutes) after receiving a blood specimen (see Blood for Emergency Transfusion, p. 36). However, a group O, Rh$_0$-negative RBC unit or units should be used when a patient's blood type is unknown with insufficient time to determine it. We stock such units (in a monitored refrigerator) in the Emergency Medicine department to facilitate such use recommending as few units as possible be infused while the patient's blood specimen collected on arrival is being typed *stat.*; then we can switch to appropriate type-specific (ABO and Rh) units. At least, ABO-identical units rather than O-negative RBC should be transfused initially if possible and, if not, as soon as

Figure 6-11 □ Form for blood component transfusion (chart and blood bank two-part copies).

COPY

TRANSFUSION FORM

SUNY HEALTH SCIENCE CENTER / BLOOD BANK
750 E. Adams St., Syracuse, NY 13210

NO.   DATE

We/I certify that before starting the transfusion the following were checked and found to be identical.

1. Patient's name and hospital number on wrist band and transfusion form.
2. Unit number, component, and unit ABO and Rh type on container and transfusion form.

NAME   LOC.

BIRTHDAY   SEX

SIGNATURE _____

RECIPIENT TYPE   DONOR TYPE

SIGNATURE _____

UNIT / POOL   EXP. DATE

DATE _____ TIME STARTED _____

COMPONENT   TECH

AMOUNT GIVEN _____ ML TIME COMPLETED _____
(IF LESS THAN AMOUNT ISSUED)

CROSSMATCH

□ Transfusion reaction occurred. Submit transfusion reaction workup.

COMMENTS

INSPECTED &
ISSUED BY: INITIALS _____ DATE _____ TIME _____

TO: _____ SIGNATURE _____

When the administration of this unit is completed, the chart copy is to be placed in the Patient's Chart.

Table 6–8 □ SOME CAUSES OF ABO GROUPING DISCF

	Forward Typing Problems
Unexpected positive reactions	Acquired B antigen associated with colon and gastric cancers, intestinal obstructions
	Cord cells contaminated with Wharton's jelly
	Autoagglutination caused by cold autoantibodies
	Cells heavily coated with warm autoantibody
	Polyagglutination
	Acriflavine antibody (against dye used in anti-B)
	Genetic chimerism*
	Bone marrow transplants*
	Transfusion reactions due to administration of red cells outside ABO group*
Unexpected negative reactions	A or B subgroups
	Antigen depression due to leukemia or other disease state
	High levels of soluble blood group substances associated with pseudomucinous ovarian cyst
	Age of patient (elderly, newborn)
	Hypogammaglobulinemia
	Immunosuppression
	Genetic chimerism

From Henry JB: Clinical Diagnosis and Management by Laboratory Methods, 19th ed. Philadelphia, WB Saunders Co, 1996, p 758.
*Look for mixed field appearance of reactions with reagent antisera.

available after typing of the patient's blood specimen (see Table 6–1). This response will conserve O-negative inventory (often marginal and labile) and lessen infusion of potentially incompatible group O plasma with reciprocal antibodies (anti-A and anti-B). Even with administration of packed RBC, a significant volume of residual plasma is infused with multiple transfusions, i.e., in a patient massively transfused. When a patient, usually with a history of prior blood transfusions, pregnancies, or major surgeries or trauma, shows an alloantibody in plasma, group O, Rh_0 (D)-negative units transfused can cause a hemolytic transfusion reaction.

Switching Blood Types

Check, the Transfusion Medicine blood product inventory periodically, especially on long weekends with holidays. Be aware of any actual or impending shortfalls; the latter may be anticipated with trauma patients and others currently receiving RBC in substantial quantities. Group O, Rh_0- negative RBC units and group AB FFP are most frequently marginal or depleted. However, it is preferable to retain, in inventory, at least two units of O-negative RBC in anticipation of a new admission or demand for a female of childbearing age or potential for pregnancy. Switching ABO and Rh_0 types may be required (see Table 6–1). Males and postmenopausal or sterile females (Rh_0 (D) negative), especially those who are elderly, can tolerate several units of group O Rh_0-positive RBC within first 24 hours and often longer before sensitization appears; by this time, the patient should be stable or the Rh_0-negative inventory should be replenished, or both.

■ MASSIVE TRANSFUSION

Massive transfusion in excess of one blood volume, or 5 liters, or 10 units, of blood in 24 hours for a 70-kg adult requires initial and follow-up information or knowledge of the patient's weight (in kilograms) with hematocrit (to calculate total blood volume at 70 mL/kg) and plasma volume (Plasmacrit = 1 − Hematocrit), plus total number and variety of specific blood components infused, prothrombin time (PT), partial thromboplastin time (PTT), fibrinogen, thrombin time (TT), and platelet count. A visit to the operating room or recovery room in direct communication with surgeons and anesthesiologists can provide most current and anticipated utilization of blood components, anticoagulants, estimated blood loss, and laboratory monitoring (see Table 6–6). Risk or evidence of a dilutional coagulopathy can be confirmed with adjustment of replacement component therapy, i.e., cryoprecipitate for fibrinogen levels below 100 mg/dL, fresh frozen plasma (FFP) for prolonged PT and PTT, and red blood cells for attainment of trigger hematocrit, i.e., ~25%, appropriate for patient's cardiopulmonary status and hemodynamic signs and symptoms, especially hypotension and tachycardia with blood gases (PO_2, O_2 saturation) (see Table 6–7). Platelet count may not reflect the need for platelet components in the presence of platelet dysfunction attributable to cardiopulmonary bypass equipment, thrombogenic surfaces, or medications. Drugs such as aprotinin, a serine protease inhibitor, provide an effective inhibitory activity on both plasmin and kallikrein with preservation of platelet adhesiveness. Desmopressin (DDAVP) also appears to make platelets more adhesive with a decrease in bleeding attributed to inducing an increase in circulating high-molecular-weight von Willebrand factor.

Replacement therapy with specific blood components is based on monitoring patient clinically and with selected laboratory measurements rather than a formula for number of RBC or other blood products infused (see Table 6–7).

Guidelines for an average-sized adult (70 kg) are 1 unit of random-donor platelets per 10 kg of body weight (about 6 to 8 pooled units or one single-donor platelet apheresis) in the presence of microvascular bleeding (diffuse oozing from multiple sites) before confirmation of thrombocytopenia or a platelet count of approximately $100,000/\mu L$ or when platelet dysfunction is suspected. For platelet counts confirmed as $50,000/\mu L$ or less, two six-pack, platelet pools or two single-donor platelet apheresis products are in order. Enumeration of a patient's platelets (counts) 10 minutes after infusion provides a guideline for continuation of appropriate platelet therapy.

Thawed FFP (p. 59) is administered in a dosage of 10 to 15 mL/kg of body weight (variable volume per unit of FFP should be noted to prescribe approximate number of FFP units for transfusion) after confirmation of coagulation factor deficiencies with PT/PTT about 1.5 times normal range of each. Subsequent PT and PTT measurements are performed periodically and as indicated by patient's clinical condition.

Volume overload may ensue with excess infusion of platelets and FFP coupled with RBC (see Table 6–7).

Cryoprecipitate units proportional to patient's degree of hypofibrinogenemia should be transfused as a thawed 6-unit pool for levels of 50 to 100 mg/dL and a thawed 12-unit cryoprecipitate (pool) for fibrinogen levels less than 50 mg/dL. Although fibrinogen is an acute-phase reactant and thus can increase in concentration within a few hours, cryoprecipitate units with a minimal volume increment may receive less attention or use than other blood products in massive transfusion replacement therapy. Repeat fibrinogen assays and thrombin time (TT) measurements are prerequisite to continuing appropriate cryoprecipitate transfusions and maintaining a fibrinogen level at or above 100 mg/dL. With timely laboratory monitoring of coagulation (Chapter 9), in association with appropriate component replacement, and bleeding control, a favorable outcome may be anticipated without depletion of the blood inventory minimal stock. Dilutional hypofibrinogenemia and thrombocytopenia are the major causes of demands on blood components, but DIC may also be observed with microvascular bleeding (slow diffuse oozing). Factor VIII, being an acute-phase reactant, usually remains above 30% minimum with factor V levels (factor V present in FFP) above 5–10% level necessary for coagulation. A patient with chronic liver disease may also require factor VII present in FFP and stored liquid plasma and vitamin K administration intravenously as an alternative and at an appropriate time.

■ INCOMPATIBLE CROSSMATCH

Nuisance Antibodies

Several situations arise when a patient's blood specimen is determined to be incompatible with any and all available units of blood in inventory and so-called nuisance antibodies have been ruled out (Table 6–9). Three occur most frequently (see below) and can be a special challenge for finding compatible blood units in a timely manner. Not only may such be difficult and time consuming but even impossible to accomplish (because of insufficient time) despite extraordinary efforts in further testing and searching for available compatible units.

Multiple Alloantibodies

Patients with multiple alloantibodies, autoantibodies, or an antibody to a high-prevalence antigen in their plasma or sera are three examples that may be encountered most frequently. In the presence of multiple erythrocyte antibodies, e.g., anti-K, anti-E, anti-Fy^a, and anti-Jk^b, the blood bank staff will type all available units of appropriate ABO type in the blood inventory to identify corresponding antigen-negative units; a regular complete crossmatch is then carried out and only compatible units are released. Regional as well as national blood supply sources and rare donor files may have to be checked when antigen-negative units are not found "on the shelf." Close communication and coordination with an attending clinician or clinicians, blood bank technologist, and outside resources are then most important, especially in an emergency situation with a hemodynamically unstable patient in critical need of blood.

When a patient has an erythrocyte alloantibody to an antigen that is present on a very high percentage of blood donor units, it will appear to be incompatible with all erythrocytes tested. Se-

Table 6–9 □ HIGH TITER, LOW AVIDITY (HTLA), Bg, AND Sid ANTIBODIES

Blood Group System or Antigen Collection	Comments	Incidence in Whites (%)
HTLA Antibodies		
Chido/Rodgers	Cha, Rga, and JMH are determinants of the C4 complement component coded for at the HLA locus, abundant in plasma	98 (Cha); 97 (Rga)
John Milton Hagen		98 (JMH)
Knops	Kna and McCa are determinants of erythrocyte complement receptor 1	99 (Kna)
McCoy		99 (McCa)
York	Yka and Csa are white cell determinants expressed on erythrocytes and in plasma	92 (Yka)
Cost-Sterling		98 (Csa)
Bg Antibodies	Bg antibodies react with HLA antigen remnants on the mature erythrocyte membrane Bga = HLA-B7 Bgb = HLA-Bw17 Bgc = HLA-A28	
Sid Antibodies	Sda antigen is abundant in urine; rare "super-Sid" erythrocytes with very strong expression of the Sda antigen exist, also known as the Cad+ phenotype. Transfusion of these cells to a recipient with anti-Sda was implicated in one transfusion reaction. Anti-Sda shows a unique mixed-field agglutination pattern of tightly packed, refractile agglutinates.	96 (Sda)

From Henry JB: Clinical Diagnosis and Management by Laboratory Methods, 19th ed. Philadelphia, WB Saunders Co, 1996, p 771.

lected representative public a[...]
antibodies of high prevaler[...]
whereas others may be asso[...]
survival; these may require ti[...]
ate donors from members of f[...]

Autoantibodies

Patients with autoantibodies[...]
all allogeneic red blood cells te[...]
shortened red blood cell surviv[...]
autoantibodies cannot be absorl[...]
existence of an alloantibody can[...]
cates and extends the time for c[...]patibility testing. In the presence
of cold autoantibodies, the thermal amplitude should be defined
and all compatibility testing performed at 37°C (Table 6–11).

Using absorbed serum for crossmatching, you may have to offer
the least incompatible unit as the most readily available option for
a patient in an emergency. For such patients, it may be preferable to
transfuse incompatible RBC units to achieve temporary or transient benefit through hemoperfusion even though RBC will not
survive normally. This may yield an unsatisfactory but necessary
outcome of an anticipated hemolytic transfusion reaction that can
be managed subsequently.

Compatibility Testing

The biologic or "*in vivo*, crossmatch and compatibility test" may
be performed as well to assess the potential of a hemolytic transfusion reaction in such patients. Infuse over about 15 minutes an
aliquot of RBC (40 to 50 mL) from the unit to be transfused and observe the patient recipient for symptoms and signs of a hemolytic
transfusion reaction (p. 90). With the appearance of such symptoms or signs, especially hypotension and fever, or if none at the
end of RBC aliquot infusion, collect a posttransfusion patient blood
specimen and examine for hemolysis in comparison with a pre-
transfusion blood sample.

Intravascular lysis of a few milliliters of RBC (~5 mL) will increase plasma hemoglobin visible on gross inspection, and that
amount may be measured at approximately 50 mg/dL of hemoglobin. In the absence of hemoglobinemia, it is safe to transfuse with a
minimal likelihood of a severe hemolytic transfusion reaction.

Incompatible Blood Unit Release

Transfusion of incompatible blood as a last resort may be required when the alternative is a patient exsanguinating to death. In
other words, it may be preferable to infuse incompatible blood, an-

Table 6–10 □ OTHER BLOOD GROUP SYSTEMS CONSISTING OF TWO KNOWN ANTITHETIC...

System	Phenotype	Frequency (%) in Whites*	Optimal Reaction Phase	Implicated	
				Hemolytic Transfusion Reaction	Hemoly... the...
Diego†	Di(a+b−)	0	AGT	Yes	Mild
	Di(a+b+)	Very rare			
	Di(a−b+)	100			
Cartwright	Yt(a+b−)	91.9	AGT	Possible	No
	Yt(a+b+)	7.9			
	Yt(a−b+)	0.2			
Dombrock	Do(a+b−)	17.2	AGT with enzymes	Yes	Mild
	Do(a+b+)	49.5			
	Do(a−b+)	33.3			
Colton	Co(a+b−)	89.3	AGT with enzymes	Yes	Mild
	Co(a+b+)	10.4			
	Co(a+b+)	0.3			
	Co(a−b−)	Very rare			
Scianna	Sc:1,−2	99.7	Most AGT; some saline	No	No
	Sc:1,2	0.3			
	Sc:−1,2	Very rare			
	Sc:−1,−2	Very rare			

AGT = antiglobulin test.
*Insufficient data for reliable calculation of frequencies in blacks.
†Diᵃ antigen has a much higher frequency in Asians and Native Americans.
Modified from Walker RH (ed): Technical Manual, 11th ed. Bethesda, MD, American Association of Blood Banks, 1993.

Table 6–11 □ DIFFERENTIATION OF COLD AGGLUTINATING ANTIBODIES

Test Erythrocytes	Antigens Present			Cold Antibody				
	H	I	i	Anti-H*	Anti-I†	Anti-i‡	Anti-IH	Anti-Pr§
O adult	+	+	−	3+	3+	0	3+	3+
O cord	+	−	+	3+	0 to +	3+	1+	3+
A₁ adult	−	+	−	1+	3+	0	1+	3+
A₂ adult	+	+	−	2+	3+	0	2+	3+

From Henry JB: Clinical Diagnosis and Management by Laboratory Methods, 19th ed. Philadelphia, WB Saunders Co, 1996, p 773.
†Associated with *Mycoplasma pneumoniae* infection; reactivity enhanced by proteases.
‡Associated with infectious mononucleosis and other forms of reticulosis.
§Pr receptors on red blood cells destroyed by proteases.

ticipate managing a hemolytic transfusion reaction, and have a live patient at the end rather than a nontransfused dead patient in the absence of compatible blood units.

■ TRANSFUSION REACTIONS (TR)

Untoward and adverse reactions to the transfusion of blood products by patients are encountered with sufficient frequency and overlapping symptoms and signs coupled with varying degrees of severity to warrant a prompt, thorough response, i.e., in accord with standard policy and procedure (p. 44) for evaluation of transfusion reactions to minimize a potentially grave outcome and serious complications or sequelae (see Fig. 1–1).

Manifestations

During transfusion, especially the first 15 to 20 minutes, careful patient monitoring is required with cessation as soon as symptoms or signs are detected. These may include the following symptoms: chills, burning with or without heat or pain at the infusion site, back or chest pain, headache, malaise, nausea, myalgia, or pruritus; the signs include coughing, wheezing, and dyspnea or shortness of breath; fever (greater or equal to 1-Celsius-degree elevation without any other apparent cause), rash, flushing of face, hypotension, hemoglobinuria, abnormal bleeding, cyanosis, jaundice, oliguria or anuria, and pulmonary edema.

■ RESPONSE AND WORK-UP SOP

The transfusion reaction notification then begins with a telephone call to the blood bank and follow-through of the SOP described previously (p. 44). With receipt of a posttransfusion blood specimen and a transfusion-reaction evaluation form or requisition (see Fig. 6–7) partially completed, the following information must be identified and if deemed necessary clarified and verified:

- Full name, hospital ID number, age, and sex of the patient
- Diagnoses or problem list, medications, and clinical management issues
- Patient location and telephone number at that site
- Blood product being transfused and amount (volume in milliliters) infused (see Fig. 6–10)
- ABO and Rh type of patient and blood product being infused

- History of prior blood-component transfusions, pregnancies, abortions, and major surgeries
- Times (2400 clock hours) at which blood transfusion was started and stopped and any other fluids infused concurrently.

Briefly describe the nature of the reaction, including salient symptoms and signs with pulse, blood pressure (systolic and diastolic and MAP [mean arterial pressure]), temperature, and respiratory rate before initiation of the transfusion, during infusion, and after the reaction or conclusion of the blood infusion.

The initial transfusion reaction workup *(stat.)* in the blood bank is according to protocol (SOP) with observations recorded on the transfusion evaluation reaction form report. Communication by the resident on call with the patient's attending physician(s)/nurse(s) including review and notation in the patient's medical record after the patient visit for clarification, additional information, and validation can be most helpful in finalizing the consultation report form within 24 hours (see Fig. 6–8) and facilitating the most expeditious management.

When a clerical check of the patient name and specimen identification including donor, ABO/Rh typing, direct antiglobulin tests, and compatibility testing (before and after transfusion) are unremarkable or conform and there is no visible hemolysis in the posttransfusion patient blood specimen, a hemolytic transfusion reaction can be ruled out. Other possible causes of the patient's symptoms and signs should then be considered with other possible transfusion reactions (Table 6–12).

Table 6–12 □ BLOOD TRANSFUSION REACTIONS, COMPLICATIONS, AND SEQUELAE

- Hemolytic transfusion reaction (HTR)
  Acute immune HTR
  Delayed immune HTR
  Acute nonimmune HTR
- Febrile nonhemolytic transfusion reaction (FNHTR)
- Allergic transfusion reaction
  General reaction
  Anaphylactic reaction
- Bacterial contamination
- TRALI (transfusion-related acute lung injury)
- Hypervolemia (circulatory overload)
- Posttransfusion purpura
- Hemosiderosis
- Graft-versus-host disease (GVHD)
  Acute GVHD
  Chronic GVHD
  Blood transfusion-associated GVHD

Acute Immune Hemolytic Transfusion Reaction (HTR)

An acute immune hemolytic transfusion reaction is the most grave and dreaded life-threatening reaction to blood transfusion that is virtually always associated with an infusion of ABO-incompatible blood into a patient, e.g., A → O, because of a clerical, computer-entry, patient or specimen identification or confirmation, labeling, or other human error. Failure to identify the patient accurately at bedside or to apply the correct label of the patient to a specimen or tube then or a donor blood bag or segment discrepancy or some combination thereof should reflect the culprit. Depending on rate and volume of blood product infused the ABO incompatibility will manifest itself as intravascular and extracellular hemolysis usually with fever with or without chills, hypotension and shock, disseminated intravascular coagulopathy (DIC), and renal failure subsequently.

Other signs and symptoms to variable degrees may also be experienced or observed: pain or burning at infusion site, malaise, back or chest pain, nausea, vomiting, flushing of skin, dyspnea or shortness of breath, hemoglobinemia and when plasma haptoglobin is saturated, hemoglobinuria and generalized bleeding or oozing (microvascular hemolysis or thrombocytopenia of DIC) at all orifices and wound sites. In an anesthetized, unconscious patient most often in the operating room, initial manifestations may include hemoglobinuria with hypotension or generalized bleeding at the surgical and venipuncture sites. The transfusion reaction investigation must include prompt comparison of donor-unit paperwork with patient (wristband) identification to prevent a second HTR in another patient with inadvertent switching of blood units and a check for another patient having blood specimen collected at or nearly the same time for laboratory tests to preclude erroneous laboratory-result reporting when there is no apparent other blood transfusion involved.

Treatment of an acute HTR whether immune or nonimmune is directed initially at overcoming DIC and correcting hypotension or shock with intravenous fluids along with diuretics to promote renal perfusion. With life-threatening bleeding from profound thrombocytopenia, appropriate platelet transfusions with other components should be considered.

Acute extravascular or intracellular hemolysis may occur with an incompatible transfusion as a result of other than an ABO erythrocyte antigen system, i.e., IgG alloantibodies in the Rh, Kell, Duffy, and Kidd systems. Although they may be serious reactions with fever, anemia, elevated serum bilirubin, and a positive direct antiglobulin test (DAT), they are not so severe as with the ABO system because complement activation and DIC usually do not occur.

The clinical response difference between immune acute intravascular or extracellular hemolysis and extravascular or intracellular hemolysis reactions is attributed to the higher amount of and earlier formation of TNF (tumor necrosis factor); this leads to the systemic response of generalized DIC, hypotension, and shock in intravascular or extracellular hemolysis.

Delayed Hemolytic Transfusion Reaction (DHTR)

IgG alloantibodies from the same blood group systems associated with extravascular and intracellular HTR with similar symptoms and signs or only a progressive drop in the patient's hematocrit represent delayed immune hemolytic transfusion reaction (DHTR). They can be attributed to an anamnestic response to renewed erythrocyte antigen exposure usually within 2 weeks. Actually they may be observed in two different forms in patients; the first is observed in chronically transfused patients with thalassemia and sickle cell disease who appear more as having acute delayed HTR within a week to 10 days, whereas the other form is observed in trauma or with a single-episode massive-transfusion-patient recipients of RBC and appears after 2 to 3 weeks or longer intervals with more subtle symptoms and signs. The latter may be missed unless patient hematocrit and hemoglobin measurements are being monitored. Both types are more profound in infants and children and in small-statured individuals with less total blood volume than in normal individuals.

Laboratory diagnosis of a DHTR (and it often stands alone) reflects the pathophysiologic characteristics with demonstration of free plasma hemoglobin, an elevated plasma LD (lactate dehydrogenase), and methemoglobin associated with a decrease in haptoglobin, hemopexin, and albumin-binding capacity but an increasing hemoglobinuria and hemosiderinuria. The DAT (direct antiglobulin test) shows positive results with mixed-field agglutination, and the patient's serum bilirubin may be increased 4 to 6 hours after initiation of blood infusion.

Acute Nonimmune Hemolytic Transfusion Reaction

Nonimmunologic damage to donor erythrocytes before or with infusion may also cause intravascular and extracellular hemolysis, which can occur if a blood unit is overheated in an improperly functioning blood warmer or frozen after being placed in an unmonitored refrigerator or left on a windowsill during winter. Such hemolysis may also take place when RBC are infused inadvertently, concurrently (through a Y-tube connection) or mixed with a hypotonic solution such as 5% dextrose in water (D_5W) and $D_5W/\frac{1}{2}$ NS. Transfusion of RBC through a small-bore needle (i.e., 21 gauge) using a blood pressure cuff can also cause hemolysis. Calcium, present in Ringer's lactate solution, can overcome the citrate anticoagulant in a unit of donor blood and cause clotting with subsequent hemolysis of the unit. Bacterial contamination of a donor unit can be associated with infusion of hemolyzed blood and endotoxic shock. Rarely, a patient receiving quinine may receive RBC from a blood donor deficient in glucose-6-phosphate dehydrogenase (G6PD); the donor RBC will then be hemolyzed. A patient with paroxysmal nocturnal hemoglobinuria (PNH) may also hemolyze an autologous unit of blood and especially when receiving a blood product containing complement. Likewise, a patient in sickle cell crisis with hypoxia in tissues may also hemolyze autologous RBC. As a result of bladder irrigation with distilled water during prostate surgery, RBC intravascular hemolysis may also be experienced. Finally, certain toxins such as those resulting from *Clostridium welchii* infection may hemolyze a patient's RBC. Hyperkalemia and cardiac arrythmia may be serious complications depending on magnitude of RBC lysis.

In these instances, it is important to visit the patient and review all aspects of illness and transfusion to identify the specific cause. The diagnosis and management are similar to those needed in acute immune HTR.

Febrile Nonhemolytic Transfusion Reaction (FNHTR)

Febrile nonhemolytic transfusion reactions are more commonly encountered in patients receiving platelet products than in those receiving packed RBC (more so in those receiving pooled random-donor platelets than in those receiving single-donor apheresis platelets). With the increasing use of leukocyte-reduced (especially prestorage leukocyte-reduced) products, FNHTRs are declining in frequency with every indication that they may disappear. However, they occur more frequently in patients who have experienced transfusions repeatedly or multiple pregnancies. FFP, plasma from platelet concentrates, and cryoprecipitate infusions may also cause FNHTR.

The mechanism has been attributed to the interaction of recipient plasma antibodies and HLA antigens on donor WBC and platelets (rarely the reverse of donor plasma antibodies against HLA on recipient WBC and platelets). Kinins or bioreactive substances (TNF, endogenous pyrogens and interleukins) generated by leukocytes increase during storage of cellular blood components; they appear to play an even greater role in causing FNHTR.

By definition, an FNHTR is associated with a temperature increase of 1 Celsius degree or greater during or shortly after a transfusion of a blood component; it may occur without or with chills, at times with severe shaking in nature. Since other symptoms and signs described previously (p. 90) may be present to variable degrees and fever may be the first sign of either a hemolytic transfusion reaction (HTR) or a bacterially contaminated unit, an immediate, extensive, and complete transfusion reaction workup is in order (see Fig. 6–7). Antipyretics administered to a patient before a blood component transfusion may prevent a FNHTR. After a patient has experienced a second FNHTR, leukocyte-reduced products are prescribed. Meperidine (Demerol) may be required for a patient experiencing severe shaking chills.

Allergic Transfusion Reaction

When documented during or shortly after a transfusion, by appearance of hives and pruritus, which may progress to a more systemic response of generalized histamine release (headache, facial flushing, hypotension, dyspnea or wheezing, vomiting, diarrhea) and also stridor and shortness of breath, the nature (usually IgE mediated) and severity of an allergic transfusion reaction can be appreciated. Appropriate clinical management response is in proportion to severity of reaction.

Diphenhydramine (25 to 50 mg oral or slow intravenous) administration in proportion to symptoms and signs may suffice. More aggressive therapy including steroids and medical support (O_2) may also be required, but the majority usually respond quickly (symptomatically) with localized urticaria that does not progress. A history of hypersensitivity may then be elicited. Since allergic reactions are not one of the symptoms or signs of an acute HTR, an extensive laboratory investigation is not necessary. Mild and limited allergic reactions that respond spontaneously or quickly to antihistamines do not have to be reported to the blood bank. Infusion of the blood product that was stopped when the reaction was first noted may be resumed with a mild allergic reaction subsiding.

With a past history of an allergic reaction, prevention can be accomplished by administration of antihistamines about 15 minutes before the transfusion or the use of washed RBC including thawed frozen deglycerolized RBC.

Anaphylactic Transfusion Reaction

Although rare, an anaphylactic transfusion reaction (ATR) may herald a catastrophic event that prompts an urgent diagnosis with appropriate management in the short term and long term. They occur suddenly after infusion of a few milliliters of blood, accompanied by acute respiratory distress, laryngeal edema, coughing, or bronchospasm and may also include flushing of skin, nausea, vomiting, and diarrhea. An ATR may be observed in an IgA-deficient patient with demonstrable potent IgG anti-IgA receiving an IgA-containing plasma product.

Immediate therapy includes epinephrine and steroids.

Prevention of subsequent episodes requires the use of washed RBC products or the use of blood components from IgA-deficient donors.

Diagnosis requires a high index of clinical suspicion, quantitative serum immunoglobulins, and, in the presence of IgA deficiency (virtual absence), a measurement of anti-IgA and possibly IgA antigen. Our immunology laboratory calls to our attention patients (usually infants and children) with profoundly depressed serum immunoglobulins; we confirm these determinations and measure anti-IgA and then, if absent, IgA antigen to confirm a deficiency. Consultation with the attending physician is necessary to pursue accordingly to rule out a congenital immunodeficiency syndrome and rarely an acquired immunodeficiency syndrome in an adult. The long-term implications for a blood bank to provide appropriate blood products for an IgA-deficient patient are substantial but essential to avoid an ATR and a fatal outcome.

Bacterial Contamination

A blood component (platelets more often than RBC) may be contaminated with bacteria that in RBC are usually cold-growing, gram-negative, endotoxin-producing organisms such as *Pseudomonas, Citrobacter freundii, Escherichia coli,* and *Yersinia enterocolitica;* the bacteria in platelet products may be either gram positive or gram negative.

The infusion of a heavily contaminated blood product causes a severe septic transfusion complication with a reaction characterized by bright red malar (facial) flushing, high fever, rigors, hypotension, tachycardia, feeling of heat subjectively, abdominal cramps, diarrhea, and shock; hemoglobinuria and DIC also occur sometimes. It is a significant cause of hemotherapy-associated morbidity and mortality.

Treatment of such a septic shock event is a medical emergency requiring appropriate antibiotics and steroids. Prestorage leukocyte reduction of blood collected may remove a small number of bacteria but not guarantee sterility or prevent bacterial contamination.

Transfusion-related Acute Lung Injury (TRALI)

Transfusion-related acute lung injury (TRALI) is a rare complication with significant mortality that appears within hours of transfusion; it is unusual in presentation with bilateral pulmonary edema in the absence of heart failure. Manifestations include acute respiratory distress, with dyspnea or labored breathing, hypoxemia, cyanosis, hypotension, fever, tachycardia, virtually no abnormal breath sounds, minimal if any rales, but diffuse pulmonary infiltrates in a chest roentgenogram. Acute respiratory distress syndrome (ARDS), pulmonary embolism or hemorrhage, circulatory overload, and bacterial contamination should be considered in the differential diagnosis.

Pathogenesis appears to be either through leukoagglutinins (granulocyte-specific antibodies) or HLA antibodies that react with recipient's WBC to produce WBC aggregates that are trapped in the pulmonary capillaries or through activation of complement components C3a or C5a, which subsequently release histamine and serotonin from tissue basophils and platelets. Such substances can directly aggregate granulocytes in the pulmonary microvascular circulation.

Clinical management promptly with cessation of transfusion should include general respiratory support and high-dose steroids. A confirmed diagnosis of TRALI can require follow-up study by blood bank staff and donor evaluation regarding the unit in question to preclude such a donor unit from precipitating a subsequent TRALI in another patient.

Hypervolemia and Circulatory Overload

Transfusion-induced circulatory overload with hypervolemia warrants cessation of blood transfusion with IV access maintained for limited fluid administration and all the usual measures invoked in the management of congestive heart failure and pulmonary edema. This may also include therapeutic phlebotomy with manual removal of plasma before reinfusion of RBC.

It is a preventable transfusion complication and not uncommon in patients presenting as a "transfusion reaction" workup for an on-call resident or attending pathologist. Manifestations include congestive heart failure during or shortly after blood transfusion in association with elevated blood pressure, tachycardia, pulmonary edema, jugular venous distension, orthopnea, dyspnea, cyanosis, pedal edema, and headache. Preexisting or underlying heart disease (valvular and hypertension) should be identified with added risk of circulatory overload or hypervolemia with hemotherapy. TRALI and preexisting congestive heart failure should also be considered in a differential diagnosis.

Posttransfusion Purpura (PTP)

Pathogenesis of PTP is analogous to a delayed hemolytic transfusion reaction (DHTR) with a patient making an alloantibody to a specific platelet antigen, usually PL^{A1}, but also to others in the transfused blood product. Diagnosis is confirmed with the identification of a platelet alloantibody in a patient who does not have the corresponding antigen on his or her own platelets. Patients show severe thrombocytopenia about a week (maybe up to 3 weeks) after the transfusion, with purpura, bleeding, and fever. Recovery of the platelet count may be 1 to 4 weeks as a self-limited event.

Treatment efficacy is difficult to assess because of spontaneous remission with time. It has included therapeutic plasma exchange over several days, IVIgG (400 to 500 mg/kg per day as a single infusion or for up to 10 days), prednisone (2 mg/kg per day up to 7 days) to recover a normal platelet count; for refractory patients with a high risk of intracerebral hemorrhage, splenectomy is reserved.

Hemosiderosis

Hemosiderosis is a sequela of hemotherapy and characterized by excess iron deposition in several organs (e.g., heart, liver) with their subsequent malfunction and is observed in patients chronically transfused with RBC, e.g., those with thalassemia. Since each unit of blood (containing 1 mg of iron per milliliter of RBC) will be associated with an infusion of 200 to 250 mg of iron, depending on the size of the individual, about 100 RBC transfusions will cause a significant excess deposition of iron. Measures to reduce the frequency and total number of transfusions in such patients coupled with desferrioxamine treatment are important.

Graft-versus-Host Disease (GVHD)

Pathogenesis occurs in transfusion of immunologically competent allogeneic T lymphocytes into an immunocompromised patient with lymphocyte deficiency or malfunction; the transplanted T lymphocytes may engraft in the host recipient's lymphoid or hematopoietic tissue and become functional. Such engrafted allogeneic T lymphocytes recognize the antigens on the host's or patient's cells as foreign and mount a cellular or humoral immune response against the host or patient, creating the graft-versus-host disease (GVHD) syndrome.

Acute GVHD syndrome is primarily a cellular cytotoxic response against the host that may be observed in severely immunosuppressed patients within 3 months of exposure to foreign transplanted or infused T lymphocytes. Manifestations include fever, generalized maculopapular rash (advancing to bullae and desquamation), profuse watery diarrhea, and hepatomegaly with elevated serum aminotransferase and bilirubin. It occurs in recipients of allogeneic bone marrow and peripheral blood progenitor cell transplants.

Chronic GVHD syndrome presents at about 3 months or longer after exposure to foreign transplanted T lymphocytes that generate both a cellular and humoral immune response against the host. It occurs most frequently in long-term survivors of allogeneic bone marrow and peripheral blood progenitor cell transplantation. Manifestations resemble the autoimmune diseases scleroderma and Sjögren syndrome; these include an erythematous rash, most prominent in the malar and palmar areas and progressing to cutaneous atrophy and sclerosis; sicca syndrome; esophageal fibrosis; elevated serum aminotransferase; restrictive and obstructive pulmonary disease; autoantibody formation; chronic anemia, leukopenia, or thrombocytopenia; arthritis and myositis.

Blood transfusion-associated GVHD. Blood transfusion-associated GVHD appears as a more aggressive acute GVHD and is observed in severely immunocompromised patients who receive regular blood components less than 30 days from the time they are exposed to infused allogeneic lymphocytes. Pancytopenia is prominent because donor cytotoxic lymphocytes react against the host recipient's bone marrow cells, with hemorrhage and infections as complications resulting in a very high mortality. One may confirm the diagnosis by finding a chimeric situation in the patient's blood through cytogenetic or HLA studies showing the transfused cell phenotype.

Prevention of transfusion-associated GVHD in susceptible patient recipients is by inactivation of the donor lymphocytes with irradiation or reducing or limiting the number of lymphocytes infused to fewer than those required to produce GVHD. The latter is not attainable after the use of 3-log leukocyte-reduction filters or after the infusion of nonfrozen plasma. Hence irradiation is used to inactivate lymphocytes in cellular blood components by a 25-Gy (2500-rad) exposure to a cesium-137 or cobalt-60 source; this prevents GVHD without significant alterations in RBC, platelets, granulocyte functions, or *in vivo* survival.

When blood recipients, who are not immunocompromised, share HLA determinants on blood donated by family members, they can develop transfusion-associated GVHD; hence, all genetically related blood donors should have their blood irradiated before transfusion into relatives.

■ Rh IMMUNE GLOBULIN (RhIG)

RhIG use may also be considered when Rh_0 (D)-positive cellular products (RBC or platelets) are given necessarily or inadvertently to Rh_0 (D)-negative females of childbearing age (or to female children). Such RhIG therapy should be initiated as soon as possible after the transfusion; it may also be given over several days when a large number of vials may be needed. Dosage is based on the estimated packed red blood cell volume of the specific component infused.

Therapy for children and adults with acute and chronic immunologic thrombocytopenic purpura employing RhIG appears to have increased recently because of its effectiveness, lesser cost, and unavailability of intravenous immunoglobulin (IVIgG). Patients must have Rh_0 (D)-positive, or D^u, blood type because it is not effective in Rh_0 (D)-negative individuals.

Adverse affects of RhIG therapy include a slight reduction in hemoglobin or hematocrit with reticulocytosis and the rare possibility of severe immune hemolytic anemia.

HEMAPHERESIS

Because hemapheresis is a consultation service, the resident on call, with appropriate backup of an on-call attending physician, responds to requests for this support as a form of emergency treatment or therapy. Although not a primary or exclusive form of treatment for any disease, therapeutic hemapheresis through plasma removal and cell removal play a critical role in several medical emergencies (Table 7–1). Therapeutic plasma exchange (TPE, also TPEx) is the most effective therapy in thrombotic thrombocytopenic purpura (TTP) and requires the most emergent response regardless of time of day or night. TPEx also provides major lifesaving support in patients with myasthenia gravis and Guillain-Barré syndrome, especially when they show bulbar involvement. Cell removal or reduction offers comparable critical support for patients with hyperleukocytosis (leukostasis) and thrombocythemia, whereas erythrocyte exchange to achieve a reduction in sickle cells can be lifesaving in sickle cell crisis, e.g., acute chest syndrome.

■ ROLE OF THE RESIDENT ON CALL

The call, or request to result in the most expeditious response, necessitates the following:

- Consultation form completed by requesting physician including patient's demographic information with weight, height, and pertinent laboratory measurements, diagnosis and medical problem list or underlying medical conditions, and all current medications with specific dosage.

**Table 7–1 □ RECOGNIZED MEDICAL EMERGENCIES
AND THERAPEUTIC HEMAPHERESIS**

Hematologic Emergencies

Sickle cell anemia	Thrombotic thrombocytopenia purpura (TTP)
Acute chest syndrome	Hemolytic uremic syndrome (HUS)
Stroke	Hyperviscosity syndrome
	Thrombocytosis (severe)

Neurologic Emergencies

Myasthenic crises	Acute Guillain-Barré syndrome*

Renal/Pulmonary Emergencies

Goodpasture syndrome

*IV IgG is also considered an effective treatment of acute Guillain-Barré.

- Patient stability including vital signs, particularly mean arterial pressure (MAP), vital capacity or tidal volume with oxygen therapy and any electrolyte or fluid or other deficits being managed, and help in deciding where procedure should be performed, i.e., current location especially if in an emergency department, critical care or intensive care unit or hemapheresis center area.
- Review patient's medical record (PMR), visit patient to explain procedure, obtain an informed consent emphasizing risks to benefit with appropriate signatures, and perform a history and physical examination for recording in PMR with your assessment and plan, including anticipated outcome, time of initial procedure with an estimate of subsequent number and frequency of procedures and approximate timing.
- Orders for further patient preparation after venous access evaluation may include a specific hemapheresis catheter with preferred location site, e.g., temporary vascular catheter in right femoral vein, specific apheresis procedure with exchange volume and replacement fluid or volume, optimal end-fluid balance range, laboratory tests before and after procedure, catheter care protocol, medications, and supplement or supplements if any, e.g., calcium. Communication with attending hemapheresis physician and hemapheresis nurse or nurses on call should be accomplished by this time to ensure their arrival in a timely manner for appropriate follow-through with participation, and further involvement and implementation of optimal procedure in an appropriate manner.

Needless to state, it is most important and a prerequisite, before you are committed to perform the procedure with selection of therapeutic hemapheresis as a management option, to establish the

diagnosis by every means available and to determine the purpose of hemapheresis and the disease category (Table 7–2). As an invasive procedure it is not without risk to patient in terms of mortality, morbidity or side effects, complications, and sequelae (Table 7–3). The severity of the patient's disease and any unstable condition are crucial in assessment. The underlying disease is a major contributor to mortality or morbidity.

Although practice guidelines are established for several diseases or disorders, they are evolving or debatable in others; this often requires dialogue, discussion, and review of current literature including Internet searches to make a final decision in a collegial manner, always in the best interest of the patient. Everything is negotiable, and we can learn from our experience—e.g., a patient in renal failure with digoxin intoxication with its narrow margin of safety despite a minimal blood level elevation, refractory to all treatment modalities including Digibind and not a candidate for a pacemaker; a nephrologist and a cardiologist can be persuasive in requesting TPEx, which subsequently improved patient's condition dramatically with two successive procedures. However, requesting physicians are almost uniformly very knowledgeable about a disease in question with its natural history though less so about the intricacies of therapeutic hemapheresis and pathophysiologic effect on the overall condition of the patient including hemodynamics (fluid volume shifts, alterations in blood constituents, etc.), and concurrent therapeutic medications and other management modalities.

■ FOLLOW-UP TO HEMAPHERESIS CONSULTATION AND REQUEST

Plasma Volume Calculation

For therapeutic plasma exchange (TPEx), the initial calculation of patient's total blood volume (70 mL/kg of body weight) is based on patient's weight (kg) multiplied by 70 mL/kg. The plasma volume is determined with patient's hematocrit measurement to calculate the plasmacrit ($1.00 -$ Hematocrit) as a percentage of total blood volume, e.g., for a 70-kg man with a hematocrit of 40%:

70-kg man $\times$ 70 mL/kg = 4900 mL of total blood volume

Plasmacrit = $1.00 -$ Hematocrit, or $1.00 - 0.40 = 0.60$

Then 0.60×4900 mL = 2940 mL of plasma as 1 plasma volume

Hemapheresis equipment technology may also offer automated calculated values of blood and plasma volumes to be used in their respective instrument or machine; these should approximate manual calculations for confirmation.

Table 7–2 □ RATIONALE FOR THERAPEUTIC HEMAPHERESIS

Disease	Category*	Abnormal Substance Removed
Plasmapheresis		
Hyperviscosity syndrome	I	Abnormal proteins
Myasthenia gravis	I	Autoantibody to acetylcholine receptor
Eaton-Lambert syndrome	I	Autoantibody to myoneural junction
Goodpasture syndrome	I	Autoantibody to basement membrane of glomeruli and lungs
Posttransfusion purpura	I	Platelet-specific antibody
Thrombotic thrombocytopenic purpura	I	Platelet-aggregating toxic factor
Acute Guillain-Barré	I	Probable autoantibody
Chronic inflammatory demyelinating polyneuropathy	II	Probable autoantibody
Multiple sclerosis	III	Possible autoantibody
Systemic vasculitis from autoimmune disease	II	Immune complexes
Rapidly progressive glomerulonephritis	II	Immune complexes
Rh isoimmunization	III	Rh_0 (D) antibodies

Condition	Category	Target
Autoimmune thrombocytopenic purpura	III	Autoantibody to platelets
Autoimmune hemolytic anemia	III	Autoantibody to RBC
Factor VIII inhibitors	I	Factor VIII antibodies
Hyperlipidemia	II	Excess lipids and abnormal lipoproteins
Protein-bound toxins (mushroom poisoning)	II	Toxin bound to plasma proteins
Renal transplant rejection	III	Combined removal of antibody and cytotoxic lymphocytes

Cytapheresis

Condition	Category	Target
Hyperleukemic leukostasis in AML or CML (blasts) greater than 100,000/µL	I	Excess myeloid blasts
Thrombocytosis	I	Excess platelets
Chronic lymphocytic leukemia	II	Abnormal lymphocytes
Sickle cell crisis	I	Sickled erythrocytes

From Henry JB: Clinical Diagnosis and Management by Laboratory Methods, 19th ed. Philadelphia, WB Saunders Co, 1996, p 815.

AML = acute myeloid leukemia; CML = chronic myeloid leukemia.

*Categories taken from Guidelines for Therapeutic Apheresis, AABB Extracorporeal Therapy Committee, American Association of Blood Banks, Bethesda, Maryland, May 1992.

Category I—Indicated as standard primary therapy.

Category II—Indicated as suggestive of efficacy and on a second-line, adjunctive basis.

Category III—Indicated as uncertain with inconclusive evidence for efficacy.

Table 7–3 □ **HEMAPHERESIS COMPLICATIONS AND SEQUELAE WITH SYMPTOMS AND SIGNS**

Associated with vascular access are hemodynamic changes, instrumentation mechanical problems, flow problems, depletion of cellular and plasma constituents (e.g., platelets; calcium, especially ionized) or reaction to replacement fluid such as ACD, albumin 5% (allergic), and infection.

Long-term catheter access

- Occlusion
- Infection/sepsis
- Vessel perforation
- Thrombosis of vessel

Bleeding at catheter site or oozing and hematoma

Risks of plasma (FFP) infusion, e.g., hepatitis and HIV

Symptoms/signs

- Nausea, vomiting, tetany, arrhythmias—low calcium caused by citrate, especially in elderly menopausal females
- Bradycardia, hypotension, seizures—vasovagal reactions, neurogenic shock
- Hypotension, tachycardia, hypertension, pulmonary edema—volume alteration, or change
- Related to infusion, ethylene oxide, angiotensin-converting enzyme (ACE) inhibitors—anaphylaxis and sepsis
- Anemia (decrease ~10–20%), thrombocytopenia (decrease ~30%), and hypofibrinogenemia (decrease ~50%), loss of blood components may be observed with procedure(s) especially in single peripheral blood progenitor cell (PBPC) 16-liter processing.

A calculated plasma volume provides an early point of departure for planning and ordering an anticipated volume of replacement fluid (5% albumin, thawed, fresh frozen, cryopoor plasma or solvent-detergent plasma for selected patients) to have on hand when the procedure is underway.

Exchange Volume and Replacement Fluid

A standard TPEx volume and volume-for-volume (V/V) replacement solution should approximate 40 to 50 mL/kg and consist of a mixture of crystalloid (normal/physiologic saline) and a colloid such as 5% albumin or plasma appropriate for the individual patient's needs and disorder. A common mixture of a replacement fluid is ⅔ colloid and ⅓ crystalloid. In elderly or unstable patients, a higher percentage (up to 100%) of colloid may be used as replacement fluid. In TTP and hemolytic uremic syndrome

(HUS), colloid (near, up to, or at 100%) in the form of cryopoor FFP, FFP, or SD plasma is about a 50–60% plasma volume replacement in a 1-volume exchange and even higher (about 65–70%) for a 1½-volume exchange. Depending on the frequency of TPExs (every day or every other day) and volume exchanged (1 to 1½ volumes) with replacement fluids as a proportion of plasma or albumin and normal saline, coagulation factor replacement may be necessary. However, fibrinogen as an acute-phase reactant will return from values as low as 50 mg/dL to greater than 100 mg/dL in the patient's plasma within several hours or overnight.

■ PRACTICE GUIDELINES

Practice guidelines as such are guidelines that may be used, modified, or not used by physicians as guidelines in their practice; *they are not and should not be construed as the standard of practice.* It is with this caution in mind that the following are offered.

Miniguidelines For Selected Diseases and Diagnoses Employing TPEx

Hematologic Disease

- TTP/HUS in adult—TPEx daily until onset of remission (subjective or objective improvement sustained with platelet number recovery, normal LD, rising trend on the hemogram); then TPEx every other day, with patient monitored closely including days not exchanged for evidence of relapse over a sufficient interval in weeks or days to attain a sustained remission (varies with patient and disease severity).
- Hyperviscosity syndrome in Waldenström's macroglobulinemia and selectively in multiple myeloma (i.e., IgM)—one or two TPEx.
- Posttransfusion purpura (PTP)—one or two TPEx to attain a hematologic remission.

Neurologic Disease

- Acute Guillain-Barré syndrome or autoimmune inflammatory demyelinating polyneuropathy—TPEx daily or every other day, until clinical improvement, particularly in patients with actual or impending respiratory failure.
- Chronic inflammatory demyelinating polyradiculopathy (CIDP)—two TPEx weekly initially for 3 or 4 weeks, subsequently once weekly, and then progressing to biweekly and monthly or longer to maintain clinical improvement objectively.

- Myasthenia gravis—TPEx initially over 3 consecutive days or every other day for a week and then once a week in long-term management.
- Paraprotein peripheral neuropathy—TPEx biweekly over 3 or 4 weeks as clinical condition warrants.

Renal Disease

- Acute renal failure (ARF) in multiple myeloma—TPEx initially daily for 1 or 2 weeks or every other day after first week as clinical condition warrants.
- Cryoglobulinemia—TPEx weekly, biweekly, or monthly as needed.
- Goodpasture syndrome—TPEx daily over 10 to 14 days or less depending on use of immunosuppressive therapy and antibody titers.
- Rapidly progressive glomerulonephritis (RPGN)—TPEx daily on average about 7 days.

Miniguidelines for Selected Diseases or Diagnoses Employing Cytapheresis or Cytoreduction

As indicated previously with TPEx, these are only guidelines that may be used, modified or not, in therapeutic hemapheresis of cytoreduction; they neither are nor intended to be standards of practice.

- Leukemia, nonlymphocytic in blast crisis—hyperleukocytosis with leukocyte counts greater than $100,000/\mu L$. Reduce count to $100,000/\mu L$ or less or a 60% reduction after first procedure. Leukostasis, cerebral or pulmonary involvement, and concurrent therapy may alter frequency and intensity of leukapheresis.
- Essential thrombocythemia—platelet counts greater than $1,000,000/\mu L$ in symptomatic patients with headache and both thrombotic and bleeding episodes, to lower count to approximate normal value especially in microvascular circulation with microinfarction potential; platelet count greater than $800,000/\mu L$ in asymptomatic patients, in anticipation of an invasive procedure, to approximate normal platelet count value.

■ VENOUS ACCESS, BLOOD FLOW, AND CATHETERS

Antecubital, femoral and subclavian veins must be adequate to tolerate a high flow rate (20 to 130 mL per minute) as whole blood flow rate (WBFR). A large-gauge needle (16 to 18 gauge) in antecubital veins (single arm or both arms) or a large stiff catheter (with double or triple lumen) usually in femoral vein are considered temporary over 2 to 3 weeks or permanent for months. Such access ensures drawing whole blood from patient with addition of antico-agulant (citrate or heparin) before it is made to flow into the hema-pheresis machine for separation and removal of specific blood con-stituent (i.e., leukocytes, platelets, plasma constituent, or plasma itself for discard) and then returning residual blood devoid of a constituent to patient; hence, reference is made to draw and re-turn lines where flow-rate problems or alterations (decline) may arise as a result of catheter positioning including against lumen, fibrin flaps or plugs, and thrombi, which may give rise to emboli. Infection at catheter-insertion site or within catheter lumen after intimal injury may also progress to sepsis and can be a serious life-threatening condition. Catheter care, including flushing an antico-agulant into the lumens per a defined protocol regularly with site examination and cleansing by hemapheresis nurses, is of the utmost importance to prevent complications and assure continu-ing access. Patient positional changes and manipulation of the catheter including replacement at another venous site may be re-quired especially with a thrombotic obstruction and urokinase as a lytic agent no longer available for use.

After completion of TPEx series, orders must be written for a special protocol of catheter removal; it may be initiated on the same or preferably the next day when the patient has a fibrinogen level of about 100 mg/dL and a platelet count of 50,000 to 100,000/μL.

■ PATIENT MONITORING CHALLENGES

If catheter-flow problems alluded to previously are number one, others less frequent and more of an inconvenience or discomfort, if not a complication that may delay procedure, are also shown in Table 7–3; citrate excess with hypocalcemia (confirmed by the pa-tient's ionized-calcium determination with symptoms as vague as nausea and specific as "tingling" about lips), hypokalemia, and hy-pomagnesemia may coexist and make replacement therapy more complex to relieve symptoms.

- Hypotension without significant heart rate increase usually re-flects a vasovagal reaction (not uncommon in patients with acute Gullain-Barré syndrome), and it is usually relieved with patient placed in the Trendelenburg position and given a bolus of fluid at hand.
- Allergic reactions (urticaria) in patients receiving large volumes of FFP with repeated TPEx are readily relieved with diphenhy-dramine (25 to 50 mg po or slow IV depending on severity of symptoms and size of patient).

After several TPEx or leukapheresis procedures for peripheral blood progenitor cell collections, patients may exhibit a drop in hematocrit or platelets, or both, that necessitate hemotherapy replacement with appropriate component to sustain minimal hematocrit ~22 to 25 and platelets of 50,000 to 100,000/µL depending on clinical condition subjectively and objectively (see Table 7–3).

■ PERIPHERAL BLOOD PROGENITOR CELL (PBPC) COLLECTIONS

Such patients are usually scheduled with autologous/autogeneic or allogeneic collections accomplished during regular work hours on weekdays. However, residents may be involved in such a patient's leukapheresis while on call when it extends over a weekend or into the evening to achieve a target cell collection of 5 to 6 × 10^6 CD34–positive cells per kilogram of body weight; 12 to 16 liters of blood are processed over 3 to 4 hours, and so the patient may experience symptoms of hypocalcemia associated with low levels of serum magnesium and potassium. Oral calcium supplementation and milk ingestion may provide relief but if persistent may require an infusion of calcium gluconate (1 g in 100 mL of normal saline) parenterally at 75 to 125 mL per hour, adjusted accordingly for symptoms of "tingling" or "tightness" in throat with or without nausea. Other complications are similar to those described previously in Table 7–3 and managed in a similar manner. These patients usually have a permanent catheter in their subclavian vein and also experience, to varying degrees, similar flow problems requiring corrective measures described with TPEx.

BASIC HEMATOLOGY

On-call responsibilities in hematology relate primarily to severe anemias, hematopoietic malignancies, and coagulopathies. Some of the laboratory tests involved in these diagnoses are routine and available round the clock in most laboratories. However the pathologist is required to interpret some diagnostic tests, including morphologic assessment of bone marrow and peripheral blood films. Evaluation of hemostasis and coagulation is often essential in providing components in hemotheraphy. Basic investigation and the approach to severe anemia are discussed in this chapter, whereas subsequent chapters address hematologic malignancies and coagulation disorders.

■ BASIC INVESTIGATIONS
AND THEIR INTERPRETATION

Basic investigations in hematology include a complete blood count (including platelet count), a differential leukocyte count, and evaluation of the peripheral blood smear. Other investigations that are usually readily available include reticulocyte count and basic coagulation studies (prothrombin time, partial thromboplastin time, and thrombin time). Based on the clinical features and results of these measurements, additional tests may be undertaken for definitive diagnosis.

Complete Blood Count (CBC)

The CBC includes:

- White blood cell count (WBC)
- Red blood cell count (RBC)
- Hemoglobin (Hb)
- Hematocrit (Hct)
- Mean cell volume (MCV)
- Mean cell hemoglobin (MCH)
- Mean cell hemoglobin concentration (MCHC)
- Red blood cell distribution width (RDW)
- Platelet count

The CBC is one of the most accessible laboratory tests, and many automated instruments based on it are available in the market. Automated instrumentation, however, is subject to certain pitfalls (Table 8–1), and the peripheral blood film morphology helps confirm CBC values. Although the platelet count is not strictly a part of the CBC, it is now routinely performed by most automated instruments and, in our department, is reported along with the CBC. CBC values are age and sex dependent, and separate reference intervals are needed for correct interpretation, particularly in the pediatric population. In addition, numerous physiologic variables can also affect CBC values.

Specimen Requirements

Blood collected in EDTA anticoagulant; specimen should be well mixed and free of clots before being tested.

WBC

Leukocyte counts can be performed manually by use of a hemacytometer or by automated instruments. The latter are more reliable than the former because a larger number of cells is counted

Table 8–1 □ POTENTIAL CAUSES OF ERRO...
WITH AUTOMATED CELL COUN...

Parameter	Causes of Spurious Increase	Causes of Spurious Decrease
WBC	Cryoglobulin, cryofibrinogen Heparin Monoclonal proteins Nucleated red cells Platelet clumping Unlysed red cells	Clotti... Smud... cells Uremia plus immunosuppressants
RBC	Cryoglobulin, cryofibrinogen Giant platelets High WBC ($>$50,000/μL)	Autoagglutination Clotting Hemolysis *(in vitro)* Microcytic red cells
Hemoglobin	Carboxyhemoglobin ($>$10%) Cryoglobulin, cryofibrinogen Hemolysis *(in vitro)* Heparin High WBC ($>$50,000/μL) Hyperbilirubinemia Lipemia Monoclonal proteins	Clotting Sulfhemoglobin (?)
Hematocrit (automated)	Cryoglobulin, cryofibrinogen Giant platelets High WBC ($>$50,000/μL) Hyperglycemia ($>$600 mg/dL)	Autoagglutination Clotting Hemolysis *(in vitro)* Microcytic red cells Excess EDTA
Hematocrit (microhematocrit)	Hyponatremia Plasma trapping	Hemolysis *(in vitro)* Hypernatremia
MCV	Autoagglutination High WBC ($>$50,000/μL) Hyperglycemia Reduced red cell deformability	Cryoglobulin, cryofibrinogen Giant platelets Hemolysis *(in vitro)* Microcytic red cells Swollen red cells
MCH	High WBC ($>$50,000/μL) Spuriously high Hgb Spuriously low RBC	Spuriously low HgB Spuriously high RBC
MCHC	Autoagglutination Clotting Hemolysis *(in vitro)* Hemolysis *(in vivo)* Spuriously high Hgb Spuriously low Hct	High WBC ($>$50,000/μL) Spuriously low Hgb Spuriously high Hct

Table continued on following page

8–1 □ POTENTIAL CAUSES OF ERRONEOUS RESULTS WITH AUTOMATED CELL COUNTERS *Continued*

Parameter	Causes of Spurious Increase	Causes of Spurious Decrease
Platelets	Cryoglobulin, cryofibrinogen	Clotting
	Hemolysis *(in vitro and in vivo)*	Giant platelets
	Microcytic red cells	Heparin
	Red cell inclusions	Platelet clumping
	White cell fragments	Platelet satellitosis

From Cornbleet J: Spurious results from automated hematology cell analyzers. Lab Med 1983; 14:509.

and dilutions are more precise and free from random error. The diluting fluid lyses erythrocytes. Errors may creep in because of partial coagulation or improper mixing of the specimen. Circulating nucleated red blood cells (nRBC, normoblasts), if present, are counted as leukocytes, and a correction must be made for their presence:

$$\text{True WBC} = \frac{\text{Measured WBC} \times 100}{100 + \text{nRBC per 100 WBC (in a differential count)}}$$

Erythrocyte Parameters

Traditionally, using manual techniques, the RBC (hemacytometer), Hb (colorimetry), and Hct (centrifugation) were directly measured, and the red blood cell indices (MCV, MCH, and MCHC) were calculated according to the following formulas (with Hct expressed as a fraction for these calculations):

$$\text{MCV (fL)} = \frac{\text{Hct} \times 1000}{\text{RBC (in millions/}\mu\text{L)}} \qquad 1 \text{ fL} = 10^{-15} \text{ L}$$

$$\text{MCH (pg)} = \frac{\text{Hb (in g/L)}}{\text{RBC (in millions/}\mu\text{L)}} \qquad 1 \text{ pg} = 10^{-12} \text{ g}$$

$$\text{MCHC (g/dL)} = \frac{\text{Hb (in g/L)}}{\text{Hct} \times 10}$$

With automated instruments, however, the MCV becomes a directly measured value in addition to the RBC and Hb, and the Hct, MCH, and MCHC are calculated. Therefore the sources of error are different by manual and automated methods.

RBC, Hb, Hct

Anemias are defined as a low blood-oxygen carrying capacity as measured by a low RBC, Hb, or Hct (as compared to reference intervals or a patient's previous values). Hb and Hct levels usually decrease synchronously (1 g/dL Hb = 3% Hct, a rough approximation), but the RBC level may not do so. An important clue to the presence of a thalassemic disorder is the presence of a high normal or elevated RBC with a decreased Hb/Hct. This clue can be masked, however, if coexisting iron deficiency is present. Hct levels are falsely elevated in dehydration, in which case a low RBC may be the only clue to an underlying anemia. Elevated Hct also occurs in primary and secondary polycythemia. Accurate measurement of total red blood cell volume requires red blood cell labeling studies with ^{51}Cr, ^{99m}Tc, or fluorescent biotin.

MCV, MCH, MCHC

MCV and MCHC correspond well to the red cell size and color as observed on peripheral blood films. The MCV can be used for the morphologic classification of anemia into microcytic, normocytic, and macrocytic types, and the MCHC can be used to define hypochromic and normochromic states. Elevated MCHC values are seen in spherocytosis (as in hereditary spherocytosis and immune hemolytic anemias). In macrocytic anemias, the MCHC may be normal or low, but the MCH is typically elevated. These indices tend to be quite stable in healthy individuals from day to day. Even in diseased states, the MCV changes very slowly. A sudden change in the MCV over a period of a day or two or a single discrepant value in a regularly tested hospitalized patient should alert the laboratory to the possibility of a specimen mix-up. Some automated analyzers produce histograms of MCV and hemoglobin content, which are useful in patients with two different red blood cell populations (status post transfusion, treated iron deficiency, dimorphic anemia) where single averaged MCV or MCHC values may be misleading.

RDW

The RDW is measured by most automated cell counters as a coefficient of variation of the MCV. It corresponds to the degree of anisocytosis seen on the peripheral blood film. The RDW is increased early in iron-deficiency anemia and is useful in distinguishing uncomplicated heterozygous thalassemia (MCV low, RDW normal) from iron deficiency (MCV normal to low, RDW high).

Platelet Count

Platelet counts may be measured manually by use of a hemacytometer and phase-contrast microscope or by automated instruments. The latter method is faster and more accurate in most instances. Platelets are identified based on their smaller size and therefore need to be distinguished from debris and fragments of cells. Spurious results are possible because of unrelated causes (see Table 8–1). In some individuals, EDTA induces platelet aggregation, which makes it impossible to determine accurate counts unless blood collected with heparin or citrate is used. When the platelet count or enumeration is very low (less than 20,000) or suspect, a peripheral blood smear examination for estimation of platelet number or a manual platelet count, or both methods, are in order. In normal individuals, platelet have a log normal-sized distribution. Most automated instruments also calculate the mean platelet volume (MPV). The MPV is normally inversely related to the platelet count. In certain conditions such as hyperthyroidism and myeloproliferative disorders, the MPV is sometimes increased.

Examination of a Peripheral Blood Film

Assessment of a well-prepared and well-stained (Wright or other Romanowsky type of stain) peripheral blood film is an essential part of an anemia workup.

Specimen Requirements

Fresh blood (by finger stick preferable) smeared immediately or blood collected with EDTA anticoagulant and smear prepared within 4 hours of collection. The examination includes:

- Differential leukocyte count
- Leukocyte number (estimate) and morphology
- Erythrocyte morphology
- Platelet number (estimate) and morphology

Differential Leukocyte Count

A well-prepared peripheral blood film with a uniform distribution of cells is essential for performing a differential leukocyte count. Even then, because of the small number of cells counted manually, considerable variation and inaccuracy is possible. Automated instruments can perform differential counts based on cell size, conductivity, cytoplasmic granules, and nuclear size and complexity. Because many more cells are counted in these instruments, precision is much better than by a visual count. Depending on the type of instrument, a "three-part" (lymphocytes, mononuclear cells, granulocytes) or a "five-part" (lymphocytes, mono-cytes, neutrophils, eosinophils, basophils) differential is generated. The latter corresponds better to the traditional classification on Romanowsky-stained films. There are also digital image-processing systems that scan Romanowsky-stained slides and identify leuko-cytes. With either methodology, cells that fall outside of set pa-rameters generate flags, which require manual interpretation of the film.

The advantages of manual examination of peripheral blood films lie in accurate identification of abnormal cells and recogni-tion of subtle morphologic changes, which may give a clue to the correct diagnosis. Identification of immature leukocytes, nucleated red blood cells, and morphologically abnormal leukocytes are the most important components.

Leukocytes

A manual estimate of leukocyte number is helpful to validate the automated count, which can be spuriously increased or decreased for several reasons. The average number of leukocytes per 50-power field is determined by a count of the number of cells in at least 10 fields in an area of good morphology. The approximate WBC can be determined as follows:

Average Number of Leukocytes per 50× Field	Estimated WBC (per μL)
0–1	0–4000
1–2	3000–7000
2–3	6000–11000
3–5	10,000–22,000
5–7	20,000–30,000
7–9+	28,000–40,000+

Alternatively, one can calculate the WBC estimate by multiply-ing the average number of leukocytes per 50× field by 3.6 (if less than 3) or 4.4 (if greater than 3). Selected causes of pathologic leukocytosis are summarized in Table 8–2.

Morphologic abnormalities such as cytoplasmic vacuolation may be produced artifactually if the peripheral smear is prepared with the use of old blood. At the same time, functional abnormali-ties of leukocytes may exist without demonstrable morphologic al-terations. However, some well-documented and clinically signifi-cant findings exist, largely related to abnormal granules and inclusions (Table 8–3).

Neutrophilic granulation can be abnormal in functional disor-ders of neutrophils. Hyposegmentation of neutrophil nuclei (pre-

Table 8–2 □ **PATHOLOGIC LEUKOCYTOSIS**

Cause	Cell Type
Allergy	Eosinophil
Brucellosis	Lymphocyte, monocyte
Convulsions	Neutrophil or lymphocyte
Drugs and poisons	
ACTH	Neutrophil
Epinephrine	
Camphor	Neutrophil and eosinophil
Copper sulfate, phosphorus	Eosinophil
Tetrachloroethane, epinephrine	Monocyte, neutrophil, and lymphocyte
Other (acetanilid, arsenicals, benzene, CO, digitalis, lead, phenacetin, turpentine, venoms)	Neutrophil
Myeloid growth factors (G-CSF, GM-CSF, M-CSF)	Neutrophil, monocyte
Hemolysis	Neutrophil
Hemorrhage	Neutrophil
Hodgkin's disease	Neutrophil, eosinophil, and monocyte
Infectious lymphocytosis	Lymphocyte
Infectious mononucleosis	Lymphocyte, atypical changes
Leukemia	Granulocyte, lymphocyte, or monocyte
Loeffler's syndrome, periarteritis nodosa, pernicious anemia	Eosinophil
Polycythemia vera	Neutrophil, eosinophil, basophil eclampsia, gout, uremia
Toxemias: diabetic acidosis, eclampsia, gout, uremia	Neutrophil
Tuberculosis	Neutrophil, eosinophil, lymphocyte, monocyte
Tumors involving:	
Marrow and serous cavities	Neutrophil and eosinophil
Ovary	Eosinophil
GI tract and liver	Neutrophil
Typhoid fever	Lymphocyte

From Henry JB: Clinical Diagnosis and Management by Laboratory Methods, 19th ed. Philadelphia, WB Saunders Co, 1996, p 573.

dominance of band-shaped nuclei and nuclei with no more than two lobes) is seen in the autosomal dominant Pelger-Huët anomaly. Similar cells can be seen in myelodysplastic syndromes, granulocytic leukemia, and some infections and after exposure to some drugs (pseudo–Pelger-Huët cells). In these cases, however, mature cells are seen in addition to the abnormal neutrophils. Hypersegmentation of neutrophils, defined as six or more nuclear lobes in any neutrophil, or five lobes in more than 5% neutrophils, is seen in megaloblastic anemias.

Table 8–3 □ ABNORMAL LEUKOCYTE MORPHOLOGY

Morphologic Abnormality	Cells Involved	Clinical Correlate	Comments
Toxic granulation—dark blue to purple, peroxidase positive, cytoplasmic granules	Neutrophils, band neutrophils, metamyelocytes	Infectious diseases, toxic conditions	May be associated with Döhle bodies, cytoplasmic vacuolation, nuclear spicules in neutrophils
Döhle bodies—small, oval, pale blue inclusions in the peripheral cytoplasm	Neutrophils	Infectious diseases, burns, aplastic anemia, administration of toxic agents	May accompany toxic granulation of neutrophils
Large, pale blue inclusions resembling Döhle bodies	Neutrophils, eosinophils, basophils, monocytes	May-Hegglin anomaly	Autosomal dominant condition with inclusions, giant platelets, and, in some persons, thrombocytopenia; blue staining of inclusions can be abolished by prior ribonuclease treatment
Numerous dense azurophilic granules resembling toxic granulation	All leukocytes	Alder-Reilly anomaly in mucopolysaccharidoses	May also be seen in healthy persons

Table continued on following page

Table 8–3 □ ABNORMAL LEUKOCYTE MORPHOLOGY *Continued*

Morphologic Abnormality	Cells Involved	Clinical Correlate	Comments
Metachromatic inclusion surrounded by clear halo	Lymphocytes, bone marrow macrophages	Mucopolysaccharidoses	Inherited deficiencies in lysosomal enzymes with abnormal storage and deposition of mucopolysaccharides; predominantly skeletal findings
Abnormally large granules	All leukocytes	Chediak-Higashi syndrome	Autosomal recessive disorder with partial albinism, photophobia, abnormal granules, and pyogenic infections

Erythrocytes

The red blood cell size can be compared to that of the nucleus of a small lymphocyte. Presence of both normochromic and hypochromic red blood cells (dimorphic anemia) is best appreciated on peripheral blood films. The presence of increased polychromatophilic cells correlates with reticulocytosis. Rouleaux formation is increased with elevated plasma fibrinogen or gamma globulins (pronounced in monoclonal gammopathy). Tables 8–4 and 8–5 provide a quick reference for abnormal erythrocyte morphology and inclusions. Agglutination of red blood cells seen with cold agglutinins should be distinguished from rouleaux. Circulating nucleated red blood cells may be seen in many conditions, such as thalassemia syndromes, erythroblastosis fetalis, megaloblastic anemias, and myelophthisic anemias. The presence of myeloid precursors in addition to circulating erythroblasts (leukoerythroblastic reaction) can be seen in space-occupying conditions of the bone marrow, such as myelofibrosis with myeloid metaplasia, leukemias, metastatic carcinoma, multiple myeloma, and

Table 8–4 □ ABNORMAL ERYTHROCYTE MORPHOLOGY

If you see . . .	Think of
Codocytes (target cells)	Iron deficiency, obstructive liver disease, thalassemia, HbC, HbD, HbE, status post splenectomy, LCAT deficiency
Macroovalocytes	Megaloblastic anemia
Macrocytes	Reticulocytosis, hypothyroidism, liver disease, alcohol abuse, refractory anemia, aplastic anemia
Schistocytes	Microangiopathic hemolytic anemia (TTP, DIC, HUS, vasculitis), prosthetic heart valves, severe burns, march anemia
Drepanocytes (sickle cells)	Sickle cell anemia, Hb SC, Hb SD, Hb S–β-thalassemia, other sickling hemoglobins
Spherocytes	Hereditary spherocytosis, immune hemolytic anemia, status post transfusion, Heinz body anemia, hypotonic dilution
Elliptocytes	Hereditary elliptocytosis, thalassemia, iron deficiency, myelophthisic anemia
Stomatocytes	Hereditary stomatocytosis, alcohol abuse, cirrhosis, obstructive liver disease
Acanthocytes	Abetalipoproteinemia, alcoholic liver disease, status post splenectomy, malabsorption
Echinocytes (crenated cells, "burr" cells)	Uremia, pyruvate kinase deficiency, stomach cancer, bleeding peptic ulcer, status post transfusion with aged blood
Dacrocytes (teardrop cells)	Myelofibrosis, myelophthisic anemia, thalassemia

Table 8–5 □ **ERYTHROCYTE INCLUSIONS**

If you see . . .	Think of
Howell-Jolly bodies (nuclear remnants)	Status post splenectomy, megaloblastic anemia, hemolytic anemia
Fine basophilic stippling	Reticulocytosis
Coarse basophilic stippling	Lead poisoning, megaloblastic anemia, thalassemia, refractory anemia
Pappenheimer bodies (iron granulations)	Status post splenectomy
Cabot rings	Megaloblastic anemia, lead poisoning

Gaucher's disease. Hypersegmentation of neutrophil nuclei is seen in megaloblastic anemias.

Platelets

It is important to verify the platelet count by an estimate on the peripheral blood film. If the platelet count is normal, there should be one platelet for every 10 to 30 erythrocytes. In an area of optimal morphology, the platelet count can be estimated as follows:

Average Number of Platelets per 100× Field	Estimated Platelet Count (per μL)
0–1	<15,000
1–3	15,000–50,000
4–7	50,000–100,000
7–9	100,000–140,000
9–15	140,000–200,000
15–25	200,000–350,000
25–33	350,000–450,000
33–40+	450,000–500,000+

Clumping of platelets as a result of activation (improper collection or anticoagulation) or antibodies may be observed, just as satellitism of platelets around leukocytes can be seen. These findings may explain spurious low platelet counts obtained with automated instruments. In normal individuals, no more than 5% of the platelets should be hypogranular or exceed 3 μm in diameter. These proportions are increased if blood films are made more than

3 hours after collection. Large platelets are also increased in patients with immune thrombocytopenia, Bernard-Soulier syndrome, myeloproliferative disorders, and myelophthisis.

Reticulocyte Count

One can obtain reticulocyte counts manually by staining peripheral blood films with supravital dyes or, more readily, with automated flow cytometric instruments. The reticulocyte count reflects the degree of effective erythropoiesis. It may be expressed as a percentage or an absolute count if the RBC is known. The reticulocyte production index (RPI) corrects for the increased maturation time of reticulocytes in the blood as a result of an accelerated release from the marrow into the blood. The maturation time varies inversely with the hematocrit as follows:

Hct (%)	Maturation Time (days)
45	1.0
35	1.5
25	2.0
15	2.5

If the RBC is known, the absolute reticulocyte count is determined as follows:

Absolute reticulocyte count = Reticulocyte count (%) $\times$ RBC

The RPI is calculated as follows:

$$RPI = \frac{\text{Patient's reticulocyte count (absolute)}}{\text{Normal reticulocyte count } (50 \times 10^9/\mu L) \times \text{Maturation time}}$$

If the RBC (and consequently the absolute reticulocyte count) is not known, the RPI is calculated as follows:

$$RPI = \frac{\text{Patient's reticulocyte count (\%)} \times \text{Patient's hematocrit}}{\text{Normal reticulocyte count (1\%)} \times \text{Normal hematocrit (0.45)} \times \text{Maturation time}}$$

The RPI is useful for determining the adequacy of the bone marrow response to the anemia—a value greater than or equal to 2 is considered adequate (as seen, e.g., in acute blood loss and hemolytic anemias), whereas a value less than 2 is considered inadequate (as seen, e.g., in hypoplastic anemias).

■ ROLE OF THE RESIDENT ON CALL

Evaluation of Anemia

Based on these findings, anemias can be classified morphologically into one of several types, and further investigations should be designed to confirm the cause.

Macrocytic anemia
  Megaloblastic anemia
    Serum vitamin B_{12}
    Serum folate
    RBC folate
    Bone marrow examination to evaluate megaloblastosis
  Nonmegaloblastic macrocytic anemia
    Evaluate other causes of macrocytosis
Microcytic hypochromic anemia (Table 8–6)
    Iron deficiency
    Thalassemia
    Anemia of chronic disorders
    Sideroblastic anemia, usually dimorphic
    Other features for distinction between iron deficiency and thalassemia

Feature	Iron Deficiency	Thalassemia
RDW (p. 110, 113)	Increased	Normal to mildly increased; greater increase with hemolysis
RBC	Decreased (may be normal or increased in iron deficiency after phlebotomy for polycythemia)	High normal or increased (may be low normal or decreased with coexisting iron deficiency)
Hb electro-phoresis	Normal distribution	Increased HbF, HbA2 May see Hb lepore, HbH, etc. in certain cases

Normocytic normochromic anemia
  Reticulocyte count and reticulocyte production index
  Inadequate bone marrow response (RPI <2)
    Ineffective erythropoiesis (includes megaloblastic anemias, thalassemias, and some refractory anemias)
    Hypoplastic and aplastic anemias
    Endocrinopathies
    Decreased erythropoietin stimulation
    Myelophthisic anemia, myelofibrosis

Table 8–6 □ LABORATORY FEATURES IN MICROCYTIC HYPOCHROMIC ANEMIAS

	Serum Iron	Serum TIBC	% Saturation	Marrow		Serum Ferritin	FEP	Hb A$_2$	Hb F
				% Sideroblasts	Iron Stores				
Iron deficiency	↓	↑	↓	↓	↓	↓	↑	N-↓	N
β-Thalassemia trait	N(↑)	N	N	N	N-↑	N-↑	N	↑	N-↑
Anemia of chronic disease	↓	N-↓	↓	↓	N-↑	N-↑	↑	N	N
Sideroblastic anemia	↑	↓	↑	↑	↑	↑	↑(↓)	N	N-↑

From Henry JB: Clinical Diagnosis and Management by Laboratory Methods, 19th ed. Philadelphia, WB Saunders Co, 1996, p 659.
TIBC = total iron-binding capacity; FEP = free erythrocyte porphyrins; ↓ = decreased; N = normal; ↑ = increased.

Bone marrow examination usually required
Adequate bone marrow response (RPI ≥ 2)
  Acute blood loss
  Hemolysis
    Direct antiglobulin (Coombs') test (DAT) positive
      Determine presence of IgG, IgM, or complement on RBC
      If antibody is present, determine specificity (if possible); evaluate for cold agglutinins
      Drug history
      HIV
    DAT negative
      Consider different possibilities based on earlier exam
      Hereditary spherocytosis
      Enzyme defects
      Heinz body anemia
      Paroxysmal nocturnal hemoglobinuria etc.

Clinically the most severe anemias are those where adequate time for compensation has not been available. Consequently, significant decreases in hemoglobin and hematocrit may be tolerated well in nutritional anemias and slow blood loss, where the anemia progresses very gradually. Sudden hemolysis or hemorrhage, on the other hand, can severely compromise patients even with small decreases in hemoglobin and hematocrit, particularly in elderly patients and those with cardiac conditions.

The most life-threatening situation is blood loss or ongoing hemolysis. In the former, support with packed RBC transfusions and definitive intervention to stop bleeding are essential for management. In the case of rapid hemolysis, it is vital to ascertain the cause. Most cases are attributable to immune mechanisms, and the DAT should be performed as early as possible. If antibody coating red blood cells is found, all efforts must be made to identify the antibody by means of elution studies in the blood bank. However, in some cases a specific identification is not possible.

Two problems arise in this setting:

- Inability to identify underlying alloantibodies. If the quantity of autoantibody is large, it may not be possible to complete absorption studies to look for alloantibodies.
- Inability to find crossmatch-compatible blood. If the specificity of the antibody cannot be determined or is against an extremely high frequency antigen, it may be difficult to rapidly provide crossmatch-compatible blood, and it may be necessary to use "least incompatible" blood. In such situations, communication with the clinician is extremely important to ensure appropriate patient management. "Least incompatible" blood should be reserved for severe decom-

pensation and life-threatening complications; medical management should be attempted first (which may include hemapheresis). With administration of "least incompatible" blood, a delayed hemolytic transfusion reaction is almost assured, and in the case of IgM antibodies with a large thermal amplitude, there is a risk of an immediate hemolytic reaction.

Review of Abnormal Peripheral Blood Films

Abnormal peripheral blood smears are often reviewed by the resident. It is important to scan the slide at a magnification of 10 first to assess the overall picture. With practice, most abnormal white cells can be picked up on a 10-power scan and the abnormality confirmed at higher magnification. If the scan is omitted, important findings may be missed (such as rare circulating blasts or nucleated red blood cells). A manual differential count may be performed if appropriate. Abnormalities of red and white cell morphology are discussed in Tables 8–3 to 8–5. Review of peripheral blood films is an excellent tool in learning and is also a good opportunity to assess the quality of blood films and stains in the laboratory.

Abnormal findings should be documented and compared with the patient's previous results and correlated with the clinical diagnosis. Often the patient's clinical diagnosis is correlated with or is confirmed by peripheral smear morphology. Any unusual findings or significant changes should be reported to the clinician.

Clinical Consultations in Hematology

Residents are often called upon to help clinicians in ordering appropriate tests, particularly in coagulation, and in interpreting their results. Coagulation tests are discussed in greater detail in Chapter 9. It is important to understand the clinical scenario and encourage appropriate and efficient utilization of laboratory services. In some instances it may be necessary to call in a technologist to perform an unusual test that is not offered as a *stat.* test. Issues involved in calling in personnel are discussed in Chapter 5.

Diagnosis of Acute Leukemia

Acute leukemia may present as a medical emergency and require immediate treatment to prevent life-threatening complications. In such cases, it is of prime importance to determine the broad category of leukemia, i.e., acute lymphoblastic leukemia or acute myelogenous (nonlymphoblastic) leukemia. At the time of initial diagnosis of acute leukemia, many ancillary studies are also required for definitive diagnosis. Specimen collection and special stains for such emergencies are discussed at length in Chapter 10. We routinely employ a multimodality approach to the diagnosis of acute leukemia, and it is the responsibility of the resident on call to coordinate the various laboratory sections involved. Residents are expected to assist in specimen collection and processing and to perform special stains as necessary for diagnosis.

DISORDERS OF COAGULATION

The approach to disorders of hemostasis and thrombosis begins with a detailed clinical history. A comprehensive history is as important as any laboratory test in this regard. At our institution, pathologists are routinely involved in obtaining histories from patients being evaluated for coagulation disorders. Using this information, a plan for laboratory testing is formulated with the patient's physician, and appropriate blood samples are obtained from the patient. This is an excellent approach, particularly in the outpatient setting, because only appropriate tests are performed (preventing overutilization of laboratory services) and the patient has to come to the hospital only once.

Coagulation tests to evaluate bleeding disorders can broadly be divided into tests of primary hemostasis and tests of secondary hemostasis. In addition, many other tests for investigation of hypercoagulable states are available. Screening tests of primary hemostasis include the platelet count and the bleeding time. Screening tests of secondary hemostasis include the prothrombin time, the activated partial thromboplastin time, and the thrombin time. Evaluation of these basic tests along with the clinical history allows formulation of a differential diagnosis and selection of further tests to arrive at a definitive diagnosis. These screening tests can usually be done around the clock and allow the physicians to make urgent therapeutic decisions. Problems of hemostasis and consequent bleeding are more commonly encountered and are discussed first, followed by a brief discussion of thrombotic disorders.

■ APPROACH TO A HEMOSTATIC PROBLEM

History

A detailed history form can be useful as a guide to obtaining necessary information. Even in the setting of an emergency call, certain clinical information is essential in addition to the results of laboratory tests. It is wise to remember that it is the patient who needs treatment, not the laboratory values.

- Demographic data including age, sex, race or ethnic background, and occupation or occupational exposures
- Details of major problems including onset (congenital or acquired), duration, severity, and aggravating or modifying factors; *always assess active bleeding*
- Details of relevant previous laboratory tests and treatments received
- Specific questions to elicit bleeding history that the patient may overlook:
  Easy or spontaneous bruising, bruising after injections
  Excessive bleeding after cuts or scratches
  Nosebleeds—quantity, frequency, evaluation of local causes, and associated factors
  Gum bleeds
  Hematuria, hematochezia, or melena
  Muscle or joint pain suggestive of hemarthrosis
  Thrombosis or thrombophlebitis
- Detailed menstrual history in women
- Prior surgical history or trauma (including dental procedures) and associated bleeding
- Prior transfusions of blood products
- For pediatric patients—bleeding from the umbilical stump or after circumcision
- Details of current medications (especially aspirin and aspirin-like drugs, which may interfere with platelet function)
- Detailed family history and any history of consanguineous marriages
- Other systemic diseases, which may have a bearing on the coagulation problem

Assessing Etiology

Hemostasis is divided into primary and secondary phases. Primary hemostasis involves platelets, von Willebrand factor, and blood vessels. Disorders of primary hemostasis generally present with petechiae, small superficial ecchymoses, persistent bleeding from superficial cuts and scratches, and oozing from puncture sites. Family history is often positive in von Willebrand disease. Secondary hemostasis involves the coagulation cascade. Disorders

of secondary hemostasis (especially single-factor deficie
erally present with deep hematomas, large superficial ecc
hemarthrosis, and delayed bleeding after trauma. Family his
characteristically positive in most cases of inherited factor defici
cies and is very useful in sex-linked disorders.

Screening Tests for Primary Hemostasis

The template bleeding time test, flawed as it is, is one of the only screening tests for overall primary hemostasis. This is an operator-dependent test that should be performed only in selected instances by well-trained personnel to obtain clinically significant and reproducible results. Clearly the bleeding time will be abnormal in patients with thrombocytopenia, those with active ongoing bleeding, and patients who have taken aspirin or aspirin-containing drugs. In such cases the result of a bleeding time test will not add any useful information. **The bleeding time is not recommended as a routine preoperative screening test, since it has been shown to have poor correlation with operative bleeding (prior bleeding history is a better indicator of operative bleeding).** Because of these concerns and because this is a labor-intensive test, it is the policy at our institution to require a pathologist's approval for all bleeding time requests during off-hours. Newer automated methods of assessing primary hemostasis are becoming available and will prove valuable in replacing the manual bleeding time test.

The platelet count and platelet morphology on blood smears also serves as a screening test for primary hemostasis. The platelet count is part of the complete blood count and has been discussed earlier in Chapter 8. Counts greater than $50,000/\mu L$ are uncommonly associated with bleeding tendencies unless there is a concomitant defect in platelet function (often seen in cardiac surgery patients after prolonged bypass). The risk for spontaneous bleeding increases with counts below $10,000/\mu L$. Assessment of platelet morphology is helpful in some disorders of platelet function.

Screening Tests for Secondary Hemostasis

Screening tests for secondary hemostasis include the prothrombin time (PT), the activated partial thromboplastin time (aPTT), and the thrombin time (TT). Knowledge of the coagulation cascade (Fig. 9–1) is essential in interpreting the results of these screening tests. The coagulation cascade in vivo differs from the factors assessed in vitro by the PT and aPTT, as indicated in Fig. 9–2.

Specimen Requirements

Blood must be collected in citrate anticoagulant and be well mixed. The specimen should be drawn from a fresh peripheral needle stick and not from an intravascular line and the volume

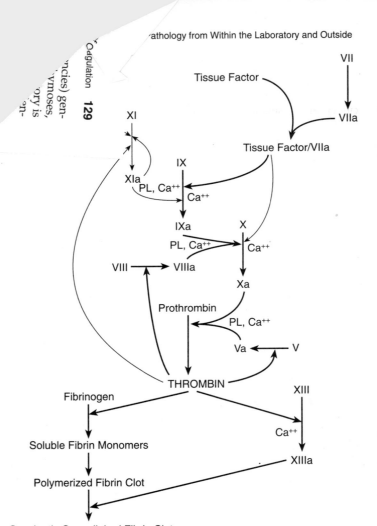

Figure 9–1 □ Coagulation pathway. *PL* represents phospholipid, which is present on the surface membranes of platelets *in vivo*. (From Henry JB: Clinical Diagnosis and Management by Laboratory Methods, 19th ed. Philadelphia, WB Saunders Co, 1996, p 721.)

should be appropriate for the amount of anticoagulant in the tube to ensure accurate dilution.

Abnormal (prolonged) PT or aPTT results must first be evaluated to distinguish factor deficiency from inhibitors of coagulation. For this purpose an equal-parts mixture of patient plasma and pooled normal plasma is prepared, and a repeat clotting time on the mixture is taken. Theoretically the 1:1 mix should correct factor deficiencies but will not be able to overcome an inhibitor of coagulation. Therefore correction of the aPTT to within 5 seconds of the control when a 1:1 mixing study is performed favors a factor deficiency, and a smaller correction or no correction favors the presence of an inhibitor. Clearly, mixing studies cannot be reliably interpreted when the initial prolongation of the clotting time is less than 5 seconds. Also, in the presence of multiple factor deficiencies, full correction may not be achieved in a mixing study.

The TT is elevated in disorders of fibrinogen and is exquisitely sensitive to the presence of heparin contamination in the specimen.

A semiquantitative assay for fibrin(ogen) split products (FSP) is helpful in the assessment of intravascular coagulation and fibrinolysis. This does not distinguish between split products of fibrinogen, monomeric fibrin, or polymerized fibrin. A more specific assay for fibrin split products is measurement of D-dimers. Typically, in disseminated intravascular coagulation, elevated FSP accompany low platelet counts, decreased fibrinogen levels, and a microangiopathic peripheral blood smear.

Based on the results of screening tests, a differential diagnosis is made, and more specific diagnostic tests are ordered (Table 9–1).

Quantitative Platelet Disorders

The causes of thrombocytopenia are listed in Table 9–2. Pseudothrombocytopenia (EDTA-induced platelet clumping) should be ruled out by review of peripheral smears and manual platelet counts, if needed.

Autoimmune immunologic thrombocytopenic purpura (ITP) is largely a clinical diagnosis and is supported by a bone marrow study demonstrating adequate megakaryocytes. Platelet-associated immunoglobulins and antiplatelet antibodies can be identified in 50–85% of cases. With newer assays, specific antibodies against platelet glycoproteins can be detected in an increasing number of patients.

Alloimmune thrombocytopenia is seen in two situations. In neonatal alloimmune thrombocytopenia, maternal antibodies against paternal antigens on fetal platelets are responsible for the thrombocytopenia. Platelet antigen typing of the parents and detection of anti-platelet antibodies in maternal serum confirm the diagnosis. Posttransfusion purpura develops within 3–14 days of transfusion of a blood product and is most often seen in multiparous women and previously transfused individuals who are homozygous for the platelet antigen PL^{A1} (HLA-A1). The mechanism is uncertain, and the diagnosis is made clinically in the appropriate setting.

Microangiopathic hemolytic anemia usually accompanies non-immune platelet destruction seen in thrombotic thrombocytopenic

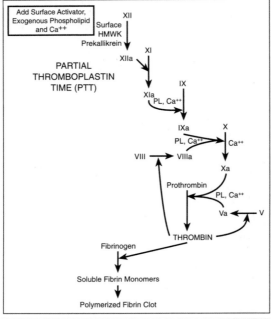

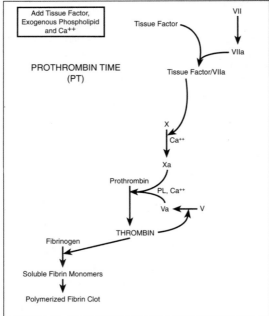

Figure 9–2 □ See legend on opposite page

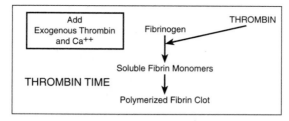

Figure 9–2 □ Coagulation screening tests. *PL* represents exogenously added phospholipid. (From Henry JB: Clinical Diagnosis and Management by Laboratory Methods, 19th ed. Philadelphia, WB Saunders Co, 1996, p 725.)

purpura, hemolytic uremic syndrome, etc. Review of the peripheral smear to demonstrate schistocytes (usually >1 per field) is useful in such cases (see Table 8–4). The differential diagnosis is made by clinical features.

Heparin-associated thrombocytopenia is seen in up to 5% of patients receiving heparin. A high index of suspicion is essential for diagnosis. Diagnosis can be supported by special studies for heparin-associated antibodies and radiolabeled serotonin secretion. These assays are valuable in guiding decisions regarding discontinuation of heparin. Patients with heparin-associated thrombocytopenia are at risk for thrombosis.

Thrombocytosis is more often secondary than primary (Table 9–3). Some cases are associated with platelet function abnormalities and can lead to bleeding disorders. Review of the peripheral smear should confirm the platelet count and exclude artifactual thrombocytosis as a result of cell fragments or debris.

Qualitative Platelet Disorders

Inherited platelet function disorders are uncommon and require platelet function studies and morphologic studies for diagnosis. Acquired disorders of platelet function are more common and are associated with drugs, myeloproliferative disorders, paraproteins, cardiopulmonary bypass, and uremia. The diagnosis is usually clinical, and bleeding time, platelet function studies, and other assays of platelet function may be useful in certain cases.

von Willebrand Disease

Von Willebrand disease (vWD) is the most common inherited bleeding disorder. It is genetically variable, and many subtypes having different clinicopathologic features are recognized (Table 9–4). Assays for von Willebrand factor (antigenic assay and ristocetin-cofactor functional assay) are required for diagnosis in

Text continued on page 139

Table 9–1 □ EVALUATION OF SCREENING TESTS OF HEMOSTASIS

Bleeding Time	Platelet Count	PT	aPTT	TT	Common Causes
↑	N	N	N	N	Vascular disorders, mild von Willebrand disease, acquired qualitative platelet disorders (uremia)
*	↑ or ↓	N	N	N	Thrombocytosis or thrombocytopenia (see Tables 9–2 and 9–3)
*	N	↑	N	N	Factor deficiency or inhibitor (factor VII), early vitamin K deficiency or warfarin therapy
*	N	N	↑	N	Factor deficiency or inhibitor (factor XII, XI, IX, VIII, prekallikrein, high-molecular-weight kininogen)
*	N	↑	↑	N	Factor deficiency or inhibitor (factor X, V, prothrombin), vitamin K deficiency or warfarin therapy, liver disease, lupus anticoagulant
*	N	↑	↑	↑	Hypofibrinogenemia, dysfibrinogenemia, primary fibrinolysis, heparin
↑↑	N	N	↑	N	von Willebrand disease
↑↑	N→↓	N↑	↑↑	N↑	Disseminated intravascular coagulation (DIC), liver disease
N	N	N	N	N	Factor XIII deficiency, mild deficiency of or heterozygous state for other coagulation factors

↑ = increased, ↓ = decreased, N = normal.
*Bleeding time in these situations is infrequently performed; it is elevated in thrombocytopenia and may be elevated in some other conditions.

Table 9–2 □ MECHANISMS UNDERLYING THROMBOCYTOPENIA

A. Disorders of production
  1. Decreased megakaryocytopoiesis
    a. Congenital disorders (Fanconi's anemia, TAR syndrome, intrauterine drugs or infection, etc.)
    b. Acquired hypoplasia (radiation, chemicals, alcohol, insecticides, drugs such as thiazides, chloramphenicol, or cancer chemotherapy, infections, lupus erythematosus, idiopathic, etc.)
  2. Ineffective platelet production
    a. Hereditary thrombocytopenia (autosomal dominant, May-Hegglin anomaly, Wiskott-Aldrich syndrome, etc.)
    b. Vitamin B_{12} or folate deficiency
    c. Other (myelodysplastic syndrome, paroxysmal nocturnal hemoglobinuria, etc.)
B. Disorders of distribution and dilution
  1. Splenic pooling (congestive, infiltrative, inflammatory, infectious, hyperplastic, neoplastic, etc.)
  2. Hypothermia
  3. Dilution by transfused stored blood
C. Disorders of destruction
  1. Combined consumption
    a. Snake venoms
    b. Tissue injury (surgical, trauma, anoxia, toxic necrosis, etc.)
    c. Obstetric complications (abruptio placentae, retained dead fetus, amniotic fluid embolism, toxemia, etc.)
    d. Neoplasms (promyelocytic leukemia, carcinoma, hemangioma, etc.)
    e. Infection (bacterial, viral, rickettsial, etc.)
    f. Intravascular hemolysis
  2. Isolated platelet consumption
    a. Thrombotic thrombocytopenic purpura
    b. Hemolytic-uremic syndrome
    c. Vasculitis (disseminated lupus erythematosus, other collagen vascular disease, bacteremia, etc.)
    d. Cardiopulmonary prostheses
  3. Immune destruction
    a. Autoimmune (acute, chronic, transplacental, secondary, etc.)
    b. Acquired immunodeficiency disorder (AIDS)
    c. Posttransfusion purpura
    d. Isoimmune neonatal purpura
    e. Drug-induced antibodies (gold, quinine, quinidine, sulfonamide derivatives, etc.)
    f. Others
D. Combination thrombocytopenia
  1. Alcoholic liver disease
  2. Lymphoproliferative disorders
  3. Cardiopulmonary bypass
  4. Others (malignancies, infection, etc.)

From Henry JB: Clinical Diagnosis and Management by Laboratory Methods, 19th ed. Philadelphia, WB Saunders Co, 1996, p 708. Modified from Burstein SA, Harker LA: *In* Bloom AL, Thomas DP (eds): Haemostasis and Thrombosis. Edinburgh, Churchill Livingstone, 1981.

Table 9–3 □ CONDITIONS IN WHICH ELEVATED PLATELET COUNTS MAY BE FOUND

Myeloproliferative disorders
  Essential (primary) thrombocythemia
  Polycythemia vera
  Chronic myelogenous leukemia
  Idiopathic myelofibrosis
Secondary thrombocytosis
  Malignant diseases, including hematologic malignancies
  Chronic inflammatory diseases, including hematologic malignancies
    Connective tissue disorders
    Inflammatory bowel disease
    Tuberculosis
    Hepatic cirrhosis
    Chronic pancreatitis
    Temporal arteritis
    Chronic pneumonitis
  Acute inflammatory disease
    Infection
    Mucocutaneous lymph node syndrome
  Acute blood loss
  Iron deficiency
  Hemolytic anemia
  Surgery
    Splenectomy
    Other surgical procedures
Response to drugs
  Vincristine
  Epinephrine
  Interleukin-1β
Response to exercise
Recovery from thrombocytopenia ("rebound")
  Withdrawal of myelosuppressive drugs, including alcohol
  Therapy for vitamin B_{12} deficiency
Prematurity
Vitamin E deficiency in infants
Miscellaneous*
  Osteoporosis, cardiac disease, renal transplant, diabetes mellitus, dry gangrene, renal failure, nephritic syndrome, pregnancy, seizures, multicentric angiofollicular lymph node hyperplasia, familial

From Henry JB: Clinical Diagnosis and Management by Laboratory Methods, 19th ed. Philadelphia, WB Saunders Co, 1996, p 709. Modified from Williams WJ: *In* Beutler E, Lichtman MA, Coller BS, Kipps TJ (eds): Williams Hematology, 5th ed. New York, McGraw-Hill, 1995, p 1361.

*Thrombocytosis has been infrequently or inconsistently reported in a variety of conditions, many of which are included here for completeness.

Table 9–4 □ DISORDERS INVOLVING VON WILLEBRAND FACTOR AND FACTOR VIII

| | | Inherited von Willebrand's Disease Subtypes | | | | |
| | | Qualitative vWF Abnormality | | | | |
	1	2A	2B	2M	2N	3
Defining attribute	vWF partial quantitative deficiency	↓HMW multimers, ↓function	↓HMW multimers, ↑function	Despite all multimers, ↓function	↓vWF affinity for factor VIII	vWF full quantitative deficiency
Commonest genetics	Autosomal dominant	Autosomal dominant	Autosomal dominant	Autosomal dominant	Autosomal dominant	Autosomal recessive
Bleeding time	Often increased	Usually increased	Usually increased	Often increased	Usually normal	Markedly increased
Platelet count	Normal	Normal	Decreased	Normal	Normal	Normal
Factor VIII	Often decreased	May be decreased	May be decreased	May be decreased	Markedly decreased	Markedly decreased
vWF antigen	Usually decreased	Usually decreased	Often decreased	Usually decreased	Usually normal	Markedly decreased
Ristocetin cofactor	Usually decreased	Decreased	Decreased	Usually decreased	Usually normal	Markedly decreased
vWF binding to platelets	Decreased	Decreased	Increased due to abnormal vWF	Decreased	Usually normal	Markedly decreased
vWF multimer pattern	Normal	HMW multimers absent	HMW multimers may be absent	Abnormal structure, but all HMW multimers present	Normal	All multimers markedly decreased
vWF binding to factor VIII	Normal	Normal	Normal	Usually normal	Markedly decreased	Presumably normal

From Henry JB: Clinical Diagnosis and Management by Laboratory Methods, 19th ed. Philadelphia, WB Saunders Co, 1996, p 734.
HMW = High molecular weight

Table continued on following page

Table 9–4 □ DISORDERS INVOLVING VON WILLEBRAND FACTOR AND FACTOR VIII *Continued*

	Hemophilia A	Platelet-type (Pseudo) vWD	Acquired vWD	Acquired Factor VIII Inhibitors
Defining attribute	Factor VIII mutations	Platelet glycoprotein Ibα mutations	Autoantibodies develop against vWF	Autoantibodies develop against factor VIII
Commonest genetics	Sex-linked	Autosomal dominant	Acquired	Acquired
Bleeding time	Usually normal	Usually increased	Often increased	Normal
Platelet count	Normal	Decreased	Usually normal	Normal
Factor VIII	Markedly decreased	May be decreased	May be decreased	Markedly decreased
vWF antigen	Normal	Often decreased	Usually decreased	Normal
Ristocetin cofactor	Normal	Decreased	Usually decreased	Normal
vWF binding to platelets	Normal	Increased due to abnormal platelet glycoprotein Ibα	Usually normal but rarely increased	Normal
vWF multimer pattern	Normal	HMW multimers absent	HMW multimers may be absent	Normal
vWF binding VIII	Usually normal	Normal	May be decreased	May be decreased to factor

addition to bleeding time, platelet count, and factor VIII:C levels. Since von Willebrand factor levels are notoriously variable (increased in response to stress, lower in persons of blood group O), repeated assays may be necessary to detect mild deficiencies. In the usual on-call setting where a patient suspected of having vWD needs urgent evaluation for surgery or other procedures, a bleeding time is very helpful as a screening test. It is important to establish the diagnosis of vWD and determine the type of vWD to select the best therapeutic alternative should bleeding occur. Classically, cryoprecipitate was the blood product of choice for vWD, since it has the highest levels of von Willebrand factor. It is rarely used in this disease at present because most patients with mild (type 1) vWD can be managed with DDAVP (desmopressin, 1-deamino-8-D-arginine-vasopressin), which stimulates vascular endothelial cells to release von Willebrand factor, raising the levels of von Willebrand factor 2- to 5-fold. For severe cases of vWD, replacement of von Willebrand factor is essential. The product of choice, however, is Humate-P, which contains adequate amounts of von Willebrand factor as well as factor VIII:C and is sterilized. Thus the infectious complications of cryoprecipitate are avoided. Patients with the platelet type of vWD need platelet transfusions to control bleeding.

Abnormalities of Coagulation Factors

Definitive diagnosis of coagulation factor deficiencies requires specific assays for the factor in question. It is important to remember that deficiencies of factor XII and prekallikrein are not associated with clinical bleeding. In a patient with an abnormal aPTT and a normal PT, assays for factors VIII, IX, and XI should be done first because they are clinically most significant. Deficiency of high-molecular-weight kininogen is rare. Isolated prolongation of the PT should prompt a factor VII assay; low factor VII may be secondary to vitamin K deficiency or warfarin therapy. Prolongations of both the PT and the aPTT signal abnormalities of factor V, factor X, prothrombin, or fibrinogen, which can then be assayed.

Distinction of dysfibrinogenemia from hypofibrinogenemia is based on antigenic and functional assays for fibrinogen. Dysfibrinogenemia is associated with a normal antigenic level and decreased functional level, whereas both are decreased in hypofibrinogenemia. If the functional assay is normal, abnormalities of fibrinogen are ruled out.

Elevations of factor VIII:C are seen in numerous inflammatory conditions and may be responsible for shortening an otherwise prolonged aPTT. This may explain anomalous results where the aPTT is normal despite deficiency of an intrinsic or common pathway factor.

Multiple Coagulation Factor Deficiencies

Several clinical scenarios are associated with simultaneous deficiencies of multiple coagulation factors. Combined deficiencies of factors V and VIII are described as an inherited trait. Vitamin K deficiency and warfarin therapy produce deficiencies of factors VII, IX, and X, prothrombin, protein C, and protein S. Factor VII deficiency usually is manifest first. Liver disease can lead to deficiencies of all clotting factors except factor VIII. An assay for factor V can therefore differentiate liver disease from pure vitamin K deficiency. However, vitamin K deficiency frequently accompanies liver disease, since vitamin K is fat soluble. The importance of distinguishing liver disease from vitamin K deficiency is that the latter can be overcome without the use of blood products (and therefore elective procedures can be postponed until factor levels normalize), whereas the former usually requires the use of fresh frozen plasma, since most causes of liver disease are not easily reversible.

Disseminated intravascular coagulation is seen in many clinical settings and is diagnosed by the presence of microangiopathic hemolytic anemia, thrombocytopenia, elevated fibrin(ogen) split products, and decreased fibrinogen levels. The PT and the aPTT are prolonged, and multiple coagulation factor deficiencies are present because of consumption. In such cases of consumptive coagulopathy, therefore, factor assays are unlikely to contribute useful information. In TTP and HUS, the platelet count is decreased, and the peripheral blood smear is microangiopathic, but the results of PT, aPTT, and TT are usually normal as are levels of fibrinogen. Elevated D-dimer levels are particularly useful in distinguishing DIC from TTP/HUS.

Inhibitors of Coagulation

Inhibitors of coagulation should be suspected when an equal-parts mixing study fails to correct an elevated aPTT to within 5 seconds of the control value. Acquired inhibitors of specific coagulation factors are uncommon causes of elevated PT or aPTT. They are found most frequently in patients with factor deficiencies and are measured by means of the Bethesda assay.

Lupus anticoagulants, so called because they prolong the aPTT and sometimes the PT, are actually associated with thrombotic tendencies and are not responsible for bleeding disorders. They are more frequent in clinical specimens than specific inhibitors of coagulation factors and can be confirmed by use of a platelet-neutralization procedure or a hexagonal-phase phospholipid assay or by demonstration of anticardiolipin antibodies. Hexagonal-phase phospholipids can overcome the inhibitory effect of lupus-like anticoagulants and thus correct the elevation of the clotting time. This assay is available on automated instruments and is very useful in quick confirmation of lupus anticoagulants. The platelet-neutralization procedure is based on a similar principle using platelet phospholipid instead of hexagonal-phase phospholipids but is more time consuming and labor intensive.

The presence of heparin should be strongly suspected when the PT, the aPTT, and particularly the TT are considerably elevated (often greater than 90 seconds). Even small quantities of heparin cause elevations of the TT. Heparin-contaminated specimens are unsuitable for coagulation tests; however, heparin can be removed from the specimen when the plasma is passed over an ion-exchange resin column (epichlorohydrin triethanolamine cellulose [Ecteola]). This procedure renders the plasma suitable for most coagulation tests and may be used when obtaining another uncontaminated sample is difficult.

■ LABORATORY EVALUATION OF THROMBOTIC DISORDERS

Evaluation of a patient with thrombosis or thrombotic tendency should include a detailed history including a family history. The most common inherited thrombotic disorders are autosomal dominant, and therefore the family history is almost always positive. Common inherited causes of thrombosis are activated protein C (APC) resistance, protein C deficiency, protein S deficiency, antithrombin III deficiency, prothrombin mutation, and homocysteinemia. Measurements of natural anticoagulants are unreliable when performed immediately after a thrombotic episode, because they are being consumed. In addition, proteins C and S are vitamin K dependent, and their levels are lowered in vitamin K deficiency and warfarin therapy. Therefore, testing for these factors is best performed when the patient is free from thromboses and is not receiving orally administered anticoagulants. Tests for the mutation in factor V (factor V Leiden) and prothrombin mutation are DNA based and therefore can be carried out at any time.

APC resistance accounts for 20–60% of patients with an inherited thrombotic tendency. This is caused most often by a mutation in factor V, which renders it relatively resistant to degradation by APC. APC resistance is detected by determinion of the ratio of the aPTT performed on the patient's sample with added APC to the aPTT performed on the patient's sample without added APC. Normal individuals have higher ratios than that of patients with APC resistance. This test is unreliable if the aPTT is abnormal to begin with. Specimens from patients taking heparin can be processed to remove heparin (see above), but specimens from patients taking warfarin are unacceptable. The most common cause of APC resistance is a specific factor V mutation (factor V Leiden), which can be detected by use of a PCR assay. Some patients with APC resistance, however, test negatively for factor V Leiden.

The most recently described inherited abnormality is the prothrombin mutation, which is estimated to be responsible for 5–10% of patients with an inherited thrombotic tendency. This is associated with elevated prothrombin levels, and the mutation can be detected by use of a DNA-based test.

Deficiencies of protein C, protein S, and antithrombin III together account for approximately 15% of cases and until recently were the only abnormalities that could be assayed in the laboratory. However, as mentioned above, their assays are unreliable unless the patient is free from an acute thrombotic event.

It is important to remember that physicians may be unaware of APC resistance and prothrombin mutation, two conditions described relatively recently. At our institution, orders for protein C, protein S, and antithrombin III levels prompt a call to the physician to discuss the newer entities (and the fact that they account for the majority of cases of thrombosis) in an ongoing educational effort.

Acquired causes of thrombotic tendency include vascular disorders, hyperviscosity, thrombocytosis, platelet dysfunction, and numerous systemic diseases, which should be evaluated clinically before extensive testing for inherited thrombotic disorders is carried out.

HEMATOPOIETIC MALIGNANCIES

A detailed knowledge of leukemias and lymphomas is, of course, mandatory for pathologists in signing out cases. This chapter aims to address the common issues that come up in the on-call setting most often. Rapid diagnosis of hematologic malignancies is essential for prompt institution of therapy. Although many patients with acute leukemia may safely tolerate a few day's delay in starting therapy, occasional cases with poor clinical status need urgent diagnosis to start chemotherapy, and the pathologist on call may be called to assist with such cases over the weekend. The diagnosis of lymphomas usually is based on examination of tissue sections, and a protocol for handling lymph node (and other hematopoietic tissue) biopsy specimens is discussed in Chapter 17.

■ ACUTE LEUKEMIAS

The classification of acute leukemias into acute lymphoblastic leukemia (ALL) and acute myeloblastic leukemia (AML) forms the foundation for selecting appropriate therapy. Although many subtypes of each exist, with extensive prognostic and therapeutic implications, the first question to be answered usually is, "Is it ALL or AML?" Clinical features may help in this distinction, but the pathologist has the last word.

Acute leukemia is defined by the presence of greater than 30% blasts in the bone marrow or peripheral blood (modified for certain subtypes of AML). The first indicator of acute leukemia often is the presence of circulating blasts in the peripheral blood. Most automated instruments capable of performing differential counts are able to detect the presence of abnormal large cells (suspected blasts), which results in the generation of caution flags and subsequent manual review of a peripheral blood film. It is customary for experienced technologists or pathologists to review abnormal peripheral films, and at our institution, this is one of the assigned tasks for the clinical pathology resident on call.

Although certain morphologic differences do exist between lymphoblasts and myeloblasts, as observed in large series, in an individual case, however, it is unwise to try to differentiate the two based on a Wright-Giemsa–stained smear alone (unless Auer rods can be demonstrated, the presence of which clearly establishes the blasts as myeloblasts).

Specimen Collection and Handling

Collection of a satisfactory bone marrow aspirate and biopsy specimen together with peripheral blood is the first crucial step in making a diagnosis of acute leukemia. Bone marrow aspiration and biopsy techniques are well described in many textbooks and are performed by the clinician or the pathologist depending on institutional policies. Although many pathologists may not be asked to perform these procedures, it is wise to be competent in the techniques, and, indeed, residency programs are being asked to provide such training to pathology residents.

Bone Marrow Aspiration and Biopsy

Indications for bone marrow studies are numerous and include assessment of bone marrow cellularity and cellular composition in hematologic disorders, staging of lymphomas and other solid tumors, and diagnosis of possible infections and storage disorders, among others. Since the procedure is invasive and uncomfortable for the patient, the clinical history should be carefully reviewed, and the purpose of the marrow examination should be clear so that adequate specimen material is collected and all appropriate studies are ordered.

A bone marrow examination is composed of two parts—the marrow aspirate and the marrow biopsy. Although in most instances both procedures are performed, in certain cases (as in some pediatric patients, patients with presumed immune thrombocytopenic purpura, and follow-up studies in patients with acute leukemia), the biopsy can safely be omitted and all diagnostic information obtained from the aspirate (and clot section). Pathologists routinely perform bone marrow aspirations and biopsies in many institutions, and it is essential to be familiar with the technique.

The site for aspiration and biopsy depends on the age of the patient and the clinical findings, but in most instances the posterior superior iliac crest and iliac spine are suitable because hematopoietic tissue persists in this region even into old age. If radiologic studies indicate patchy involvement of the marrow space (as in multiple myeloma), every effort should be made to sample an involved site, and the procedure may have to be performed by an interventional radiologist or surgeon in that case. The sternum is more easily accessible for aspiration but is unsuitable for biopsies, and sternal aspiration has more serious potential complications. In infants with incompletely ossified iliac bones, the anterior tibia may be used. The decision to perform unilateral or bilateral biopsies depends on the indication; in general, bilateral biopsies have higher positive yields in staging procedures for lymphoma and solid tumors. Bilateral aspiration is generally not necessary, unless one side is particularly unsatisfactory. The procedure described subsequently is employed for routine iliac aspiration and biopsy.

Informed Consent

Informed consent must be obtained, as for any other invasive procedure. Most patients tolerate these procedures well, and the only aftereffects are soreness at the puncture site for a short time. However, the potential for hematoma formation or infection does exist (though is minimal in experienced hands) and should be communicated to the patient. The consent form should be signed by the patient, a witness, and the person obtaining the consent, usually the physician performing the procedure. This is also a good time to obtain a brief history from the patient and specifically to ask about any allergies to lidocaine or other anesthetic to be used in the procedure and any significant bleeding tendencies. Although most patients with thrombocytopenia can tolerate the procedure fairly well, hemophilia and related clotting disorders are relative contraindications to bone marrow aspiration and biopsy.

Patient Preparation

The patient should be asked to remove his or her clothes and lie on the side or in a prone position with a pillow or rolled-up blanket under the abdomen and pelvis. The purpose is to have easy access to the iliac crest and spine on the side on which the procedure is to be performed. For bilateral biopsies, the physician should be able to access the patient from either side of the bed for ease of manipulation. The iliac spine and crest are palpated and may be marked with a marking pen or by an impression made in the skin with the cap of a pen. The area is then cleaned, usually twice, with an antiseptic solution. Under aseptic conditions, the patient is draped leaving the marked area exposed. The site is then anesthetized by means of a local anesthetic such as 1% lidocaine, with assurance that the periosteum as well as the soft tissue are infiltrated. The skin should be infiltrated first and then the needle advanced until it contacts the bone; an anesthetic should be infiltrated in a circular region of the periosteum because this is the most sensitive area.

Bone Marrow Aspiration

Many different needles are available for marrow application. It is essential to use a needle long enough to reach the marrow space (a manipulation that may be difficult in obese patients). Needles with stylets fixed by a locking mechanism are easier to use. The needle, usually 18 gauge, with a stylet is inserted over the iliac crest or spine by use of two fingers of the other hand for guidance. It is advanced until the bone is reached and then is pushed into the bone with a rotating motion. Entry into the marrow space is felt as a sudden reduction in resistance ("give"). The needle should be firmly anchored in place at this time by the bony cortex, and such anchoring should be ascertained because a misleading sense of "give" may be felt in patients with scarring. The stylet is then removed, and a 10- or 20-mL syringe is attached to the needle hub. The plunger of the syringe is pulled back vigorously to loosen and aspirate the marrow, but no more than 0.2 to 0.5 mL of marrow should actually be aspirated to minimize contamination with peripheral blood. This aspiration is accompanied by an unpleasant sensation, and the patient should be warned before the plunger is pulled. The syringe is then handed to an assistant who will prepare slides (see subsequent sections). The hub of the needle should be covered with a gloved finger or another syringe attached until the quality of the aspirate is established. Additional syringes are used to collect specimen material for ancillary studies. These additional specimens are necessarily diluted by peripheral blood, since the first procedure induces bleeding into the marrow space, and are therefore suboptimal for morphologic evaluation. If marrow cannot be aspirated (a situation known as "dry tap"), a larger syringe may be used for additional suction, or the pathologist may have to rely on touch imprints of the marrow biopsy for morphologic evaluation. The stylet is reinserted into the needle after aspiration, and the needle is withdrawn. Pressure should be applied to the area to secure hemostasis.

Bone Marrow Biopsy

The bone marrow biopsy should be performed at a different site (within the same anesthetized area) to prevent aspiration artifact (which occurs when bony trabeculae from the area of aspiration are biopsied and show fresh blood without any hematopoietic elements). A small skin incision is helpful because the biopsy needle has a large bore. The needle with stylet is advanced into the bone, and then the stylet is removed. The needle is then advanced with slight rotatory motion up to 3 cm into the marrow space, depending on patient size. It is then rotated three or four times clockwise and counterclockwise to loosen the piece of bone and is then pushed an additional few millimeters in to break the attachments of the biopsy specimen to the rest of the bone. The hub of the needle is covered with the gloved thumb, and the needle is withdrawn with lateral movements. Strong pressure is applied to the site for hemostasis. The biopsy sample is removed from the hub end of the needle by means of the stylet or other blunt guiding tool for the purpose and placed on a glass slide for making touch imprints.

Patient Instructions

The area of the procedure should be kept under pressure for at least 5 minutes and then thoroughly cleaned. An adhesive pressure bandage is then applied. The patient should be allowed to sit up after a few minutes and observed for at least 15 minutes before leaving. The patient is instructed to keep the area dry for a few days and to report any abnormal bleeding to his or her primary physician or to seek attention in the emergency department. The site of aspiration and biopsy is sore for a few days, and the patient may take acetaminophen for pain relief *but not aspirin*.

Specimen Handling

The pathologist should be able to assist the clinician obtaining the bone marrow sample and ensure that appropriate slides are prepared and specimens collected for all essential studies. Cytogenetic analysis and analysis of cell surface markers by flow cytometry have become a routine part of the examination of acute leukemias. Additionally, specimens may be required for other molecular pathology tests and for outside review if the patient is likely to participate in a clinical trial.

Bone Marrow Aspirate

MORPHOLOGIC STUDIES.   Bone marrow aspiration is performed first, and the first few drops of marrow (less than 1 mL) should be aspirated into a syringe and used for preparing slides for Wright-Giemsa staining. The specimen is then expelled onto a petri dish or slide that is tilted to allow the blood to run off, leaving bone marrow particles for smear preparation. Routinely 10 to 12 slides should be made by means of either the "push" technique (analogous to making peripheral blood smears) or the "crush" technique, wherein bone marrow particles are gently compressed between two glass slides that are then pulled apart. It is important to prepare the slides quickly to prevent the marrow from clotting. The slides should be allowed to air dry. The presence of particles determines an adequate sample; if particles are not seen, the physician should be informed that the sample may be suboptimal, and a repeat aspirate may be needed. (The absence of particles does not automatically make a sample unsatisfactory, however, since marrow fibrosis, greatly increased cellularity, and other conditions can cause this.) The remaining aspirate, after preparation of the slides, is allowed to clot and then placed in a fixative (as described subsequently for the biopsy). This is then used for preparing histologic sections ("clot sections"), which provide information similar to the biopsy and may be the only histologic sections available in pediatric patients in whom bone marrow biopsies are infrequently performed.

CYTOGENETIC STUDIES. Additional bone marrow is then collected for ancillary studies. One to 2 mL of marrow submitted in sodium heparin anticoagulant is sufficient for routine karyotypic analysis. The marrow and anticoagulant should be thoroughly mixed to prevent the formation of small clots. We routinely collect marrow in two pediatric-sized heparinized tubes (used for collecting blood) for this purpose; one tube is used by our cytogenetics laboratory, and the second tube is available for sending out to a review center if the patient is placed on a protocol. The specimen should be sent to the cytogenetics laboratory promptly for processing. If a delay is anticipated, the specimen should be kept at room temperature. Most cytogenetics laboratories process specimens 7 days a week to avoid cell loss.

FLOW CYTOMETRIC STUDIES. Marrow aspirate is similarly collected in heparin and mixed thoroughly for flow cytometric studies. The volume required depends on the cellularity of the specimen, and generally two pediatric heparinized tubes are sufficient. This is subsequently transferred to a tissue culture medium such as RPMI1640 (diluted 1:2) and stored at room temperature until being further processed.

MICROBIOLOGIC STUDIES. Fresh marrow should be collected in a sterile container or other transport medium for microbiologic tests, as needed.

ADDITIONAL STUDIES. Marrow collected in heparin or EDTA can be kept for sending out for additional studies. For DNA-based molecular tests, EDTA is the preferred anticoagulant.

Bone Marrow Biopsy

TOUCH IMPRINTS. Touch imprints are prepared by rolling the biopsy core on a glass slide; a needle can be used for this purpose. Five to 10 imprints should be made and are then allowed to air dry. Touch imprints should reflect findings in the marrow aspirate and are stained in the same fashion. They are particularly useful in detecting tumor cells in the bone marrow and in assessing bone marrow cellular composition in patients with an unsatisfactory ("dry") aspirate.

MORPHOLOGIC STUDIES. The biopsy core should be handled in the same way as other hematopoietic tissue, with fixation in B5 (or other fixative to enhance nuclear morphology) followed by formalin or alcohol fixation. Prepare fresh B5 solution by mixing B5 stock solution and 37% formaldehyde in a 9:1 ratio. Tissue should be fixed in B5 for 2 hours; overfixation is detrimental to tissue morphology. The biopsy is then transferred into 10% formalin or 70% ethanol and subsequently processed by the histology laboratory after decalcification. Excessive exposure to decalcification reagents should be avoided to preserve morphology and immunoreactivity, should immunohistochemical stains be required. The aspirate clot is handled in the same way, except that decalcification is not required.

OTHER STUDIES.   Portions of the biopsy can be submitted fresh for molecular tests or flash frozen at $-70°C$ for future use.

Peripheral Blood.   Peripheral blood must be collected at the time of the bone marrow procedure for preparation of blood smears, a complete blood count, and a differential leukocyte count. Cytogenetic and flow cytometric studies may also be performed on peripheral blood, if needed.

Wright-Giemsa Stain

The Wright stain, or Wright-Giemsa stain, is the standard method for examining air-dried blood and bone marrow films. Automated stainers are used in most large laboratories and are satisfactory for blood smears. Since bone marrow smears tend to be of variable thickness, manual staining is often superior for morphologic evaluation. The procedure is as follows:

- Place the slides on a level staining rack.
- Flood each slide with absolute methanol for a few seconds—approximately 10 seconds for blood films and 30 seconds for bone marrow films.
- Tilt each slide to drain off excess methanol.
- Flood each slide with Wright stain to completely cover the slide. Leave this for 5 to 10 minutes (staining time varies with each batch of stain used, and each laboratory has an optimal time for this step).
- Without removing the Wright stain, carefully add an equal volume of buffer dropwise on the slide. A metallic sheen should form on the top of the mixture. Leave this for 25 to 30 minutes (longer for bone marrow specimens).
- Keeping the slides horizontal, wash with tap water. Rinse thoroughly under running tap water.
- Wipe off excess stain from the back of the slides with a piece of gauze and set them vertically in a drying rack.
- Coverslip slides when completely dry.

Examination of the peripheral smear is discussed in Chapter 8. A differential count on the bone marrow aspirate or touch imprint slides should allow a diagnosis of acute leukemia.

Peroxidase Stain

The basic distinction between ALL and AML is the presence of myeloperoxidase activity in blasts. The presence of 3% or more blasts positive for myeloperoxidase or Sudan black B establishes a diagnosis of AML (except for certain subtypes, discussed subsequently). The only other definite feature of AML is the presence of Auer rods in neoplastic cells, which are found in a subset of AML cases. A stain for myeloperoxidase is often required on an emergent basis to decide the course of therapy. The 3,3'-diaminobenzidine (DAB) method for demonstrating myeloperoxidase activity is used in our institution and is performed as follows:

- Label patient and control slides. Any slide with adequate myeloid precursors is satisfactory as a control.
- Set up 7 Coplin jars and label them as follows:
  DAB fix
  NaCl
  DAB
  TRIS buffer (pH 7.6)
  $CuSO_4$
  NaCl
  Hematoxylin

DAB is available as a powder or tablet. Mix DAB in TRIS buffer (25 mg of DAB in 50 mL of TRIS buffer) and to this add 0.1 mL of 1% hydrogen peroxide. DAB is carcinogenic and should be handled carefully under a safety hood.

- Fill the other Coplin jars with the appropriate reagents.
- Run the slides through the staining procedure for the times given below, moving slides from one reagent to the next without delay.
  DAB fix, 1 min
  NaCl rinse, 1 min
  TRIS HCl rinse, 1 min
  $CuSO_4$ immerse, 2 min
  NaCl rinse, 1 min
  Tap water rinse, 1 min
  Hematoxylin counterstain, 5–10 min
  Tap water rinse
- Air dry slides and coverslip.
- Dispose the reagents appropriately: DAB fixative, $CuSO_4$, and hematoxylin may be reused; NaCl and TRIS buffer may be poured down the drain; DAB waste should be stored for appropriate disposal.
- Check to make sure the control slide is satisfactory.

Myeloblasts are recognized by nuclear features and show distinct brown granules of peroxidase activity.

Further subclassification of ALL and AML follows the French-American-British (FAB) scheme, outlined in Tables 10–1 and 10–2 and Fig. 10–1. Although important prognostically, this subclassifi-

Table 10–1 □ FRENCH-AMERICAN-BRITISH (FAB) CLASSIFICATION OF THE ACUTE LYMPHOBLASTIC LEUKEMIAS (L)

Cytology	L1	L2	L3
Size	Small	Large	Large and homogeneous
Chromatin	Homogeneous	Variable	Finely stippled
Shape	Regular	Irregular	Oval to round
Nucleoli	Rare	Present	1–3
Cytoplasm	Scanty	Moderate	Moderate
Basophilia	Moderate	Variable	Intense

From Bennett JM, et al: Br J Haematol 1976; 33:451. Blackwell Scientific Publications, Ltd., Oxford.

cation usually does not affect initial therapy. AML-M6 is recognized by the presence of greater than 50% erythroid precursors and greater than 30% blasts among nonerythroid cells. Blasts of AML-M0 are peroxidase negative by definition, and those of AML-M5 and M7 are often so as well. AML-M5 is recognized by the presence of abundant monoblasts and promonocytes, which can usually be recognized by use of Wright-Giemsa stain. For the diagnosis of AML-M0 and M7, demonstration of myeloid antigens and megakaryocytic markers by immunologic techniques is required and is accomplished most efficiently by flow cytometry (discussed subsequently).

ALL-L1 and L2 probably are no different prognostically. ALL-L2 is important to recognize, however, because L2 lymphoblasts resemble myeloblasts and an erroneous diagnosis may be made if a stain for peroxidase activity is not performed. The important pathologic prognostic indicators in ALL are immunophenotype and cytogenetics. Although ALL-L3 is distinctive morphologically, recognition of a B-cell phenotype by flow cytometry assists in this diagnosis.

Immunophenotype in Acute Leukemia

Table 10–3 summarizes immunophenotypic findings in ALL. B-cell ALL (usually of FAB-L3 morphology) is distinguished by the presence of surface immunoglobulin, with light-chain restriction. The role of immunophenotyping in AML is less important than in ALL, except in certain subtypes, as mentioned above. AML-M0 is characterized by the presence of at least one myeloid-specific marker (CD13, 14, 15, or 33) and the absence of lymphoid markers. Demonstration of platelet or megakaryocyte markers CD41 and 61 is useful in the diagnosis of AML-M7. The use of flow cytometric panels is discussed subsequently.

Text continued on page 157

Table 10–2 □ FRENCH-AMERICAN-BRITISH (FAB) CLASSIFICATION OF THE ACUTE MYELOID LEUKEMIAS

Subtype	Criteria	Approximate Percentage of Cases
M0: Myeloblastic with minimal differentiation	≥30% of ANC are Type I blast <3% of blasts are Px/SBB positive ≥20% of blasts are positive for myeloid-associated antigens while negative for lymphoid antigens	—
M1: Myeloblastic without maturation	≥30% of ANC are Type I and Type II blasts ≥90% of NEC are blasts ≥3% of blasts are Px/SBB positive	20
M2: Myeloblastic with maturation	≥30% of ANC are Type I and Type II blasts <90% of NEC are blasts ≥10% of NEC are promyelocytes or more mature granulocytes <20% of NEC are of monocytic lineage Usually >85% of blasts are positive for SBB/Px/CAE	30
M3: Promyelocytic, hypergranular	≥30% blasts and abnormal hypergranular promyelocytes Auer rods and multiple Auer rods Usually >85% of leukemic cells are positive for SBB/Px/CAE	12
M3V: Promyelocytic, microgranular	≥30% blasts and abnormal microgranular promyelocytes Rare hypergranular promyelocytes Rare Auer rods and multiple Auer rods Usually >85% of leukemic cells are positive for SBB/Px/CAE	4
M4: Myelomonocytic	≥30% of ANC are Type I and Type II blasts Percentage of myeloblasts, promyelocytes, myelocytes, and later granulocytes is ≥30% <80% NEC are monoblasts, promonocytes, or monocytes >20% of blasts are positive for SBB/Px/CAE >20% of blasts are positive for αNAE, αNBE	12

M4E: Myelomonocytic with eosinophilia	Same as M4 plus abnormal eosinophilia Eosinophils with large abnormal basophilic granules; eosinophilic granules are often PAS positive, eosinophils are often CAE positive	4
M5A: Monocytic, poorly differentiated	≥30% of ANC are blasts ≥80% of NEC are monoblasts, promonocytes, or monocytes ≥80% of monocytic cells are monoblasts <20% of leukemic cells are CAE positive ≥80% of leukemic cells are αNAE, αNBE positive	12
M5B: Monocytic, differentiated	≥30% of ANC are blasts ≥80% of NEC are monoblasts, promonocytes, or monocytes <80% of monocytic cells are monoblasts <20% of leukemic cells are CAE positive ≥80% of leukemic cells are αNAE, αNBE positive	3
M6: Erythroleukemia	≥50% ANC are erythroblasts ≥30% NEC are blasts Many erythroid precursor cells are PAS positive	3
M7: Megakaryoblastic	≥30% of ANC are megakaryoblasts or leukemic cells Leukemic cells are platelet peroxidase positive on electron microscopy or positive for glycoproteins Ib or IIb/IIIa as demonstrated by immunocytochemical methods	<1

ANC = all nucleated cells; NEC = nonerythroid cells; SBB = Sudan black B; Px = myeloperoxidase; CAE = ASD chloroacetate esterase; αNAE = α-naphthyl acetate esterase; αNBE = α-naphthyl butyrate esterase; PAS = periodic acid–Schiff.

From Bennett JM, Catovsky D, Daniel M, Flandrin G, Galton DAG, Gralnick HR, Sultan C: Criteria for the diagnosis of acute leukemia of megakaryocyte lineage (M7). Ann Intern Med 1985; 103:460; and proposed revised criteria for the classification of acute myeloid leukemia. Ann Intern Med 1985; 103:620.

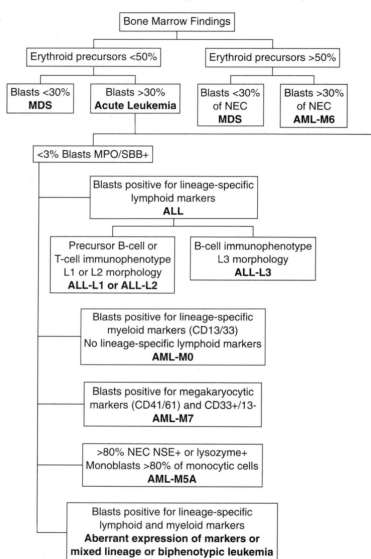

Figure 10–1 □ Classification of acute leukemia.

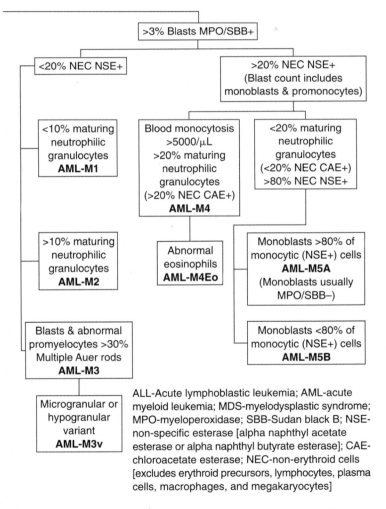

>3% Blasts MPO/SBB+

<20% NEC NSE+

>20% NEC NSE+
(Blast count includes
monoblasts & promonocytes)

<10% maturing
neutrophilic
granulocytes
AML-M1

Blood monocytosis
>5000/μL
>20% maturing
neutrophilic
granulocytes
(>20% NEC CAE+)
AML-M4

<20% maturing
neutrophilic
granulocytes
(<20% NEC CAE+)
>80% NEC NSE+

>10% maturing
neutrophilic
granulocytes
AML-M2

Abnormal
eosinophils
AML-M4Eo

Monoblasts >80% of
monocytic (NSE+) cells
AML-M5A
(Monoblasts usually
MPO/SBB–)

Blasts & abnormal
promyelocytes >30%
Multiple Auer rods
AML-M3

Monoblasts <80% of
monocytic (NSE+) cells
AML-M5B

Microgranular or
hypogranular
variant
AML-M3v

ALL-Acute lymphoblastic leukemia; AML-acute
myeloid leukemia; MDS-myelodysplastic syndrome;
MPO-myeloperoxidase; SBB-Sudan black B; NSE-
non-specific esterase [alpha naphthyl acetate
esterase or alpha naphthyl butyrate esterase]; CAE-
chloroacetate esterase; NEC-non-erythroid cells
[excludes erythroid precursors, lymphocytes, plasma
cells, macrophages, and megakaryocytes]

Based on the FAB criteria and recommendations in Armed Forces Institute of Pathology:
Atlas of Tumor Pathology—Tumors of the Bone Marrow, Washington, D.C., Universities
Associated for Research and Education in Pathology,1967–<1984-   >.

Table 10-3 □ IMMUNOPHENOTYPIC CLASSIFICATION OF ACUTE LYMPHOBLASTIC LEUKEMIA (ALL)

Subsets of ALL	Immunophenotype											Approximate Percentage of Population
	Tdt	DR	CD2	CD5	CD10	CD19	CD20	CD24	SIg	CIg		
T cell	+	−	+	+	−	−	−	−	−	−		10–20
Early pre-B	+	+	−	−	+	+	−	+	−	−		60–70
Pre-B	+	+	−	−	+	+	+	+	−	+		15–20
B cell	−	+	−	−	−	+	+	+	+	−		1–3

Tdt = terminal deoxynucleotidyl transferase
DR = HLA-DR histocompatibility antigen
CD = cluster designation: CD2 and CD5, pan–T cell; CD10, common ALL; CD19, CD20, CD24, pan–B cell
SIg = surface immunoglobulin
CIg = cytoplasmic immunoglobulin

Cytogenetics in Acute Leukemia

Common cytogenetic abnormalities associated with acute leukemias are listed in Table 14–2.

■ OTHER HEMATOPOIETIC MALIGNANCIES

Handling of lymph nodes and other hematopoietic tissues (e.g., spleen) is discussed in Chapter 17. Specimens should be divided for different studies and handled appropriately. On-call issues in such cases usually revolve around classification based on flow cytometric studies, since that is one of the few tests that can be performed on a *stat.* basis. Our laboratory uses gated two-color flow cytometric analysis, though multicolor analysis is becoming the norm. To facilitate the selection of surface markers to be tested, we have developed panels for use in general categories of neoplasms. For instance, the acute leukemia panel, which is used for ALL and AML, consists of the following pairs of antigens: CD7/CD2, CD4/CD8, CD20/CD5, CD10/CD19, kappa/lambda, CD3/CD16+56, CD41/CD13, glycophorin/CD14, CD15/CD33, and CD34/CD1. The use of predetermined panels is helpful in expediting specimen setup for flow cytometric analysis.

The expected (usual) immunophenotypes of some common lymphoproliferative disorders are listed below. These are based on the revised European-American lymphoma (REAL) classification.

- B-cell chronic lymphocytic leukemia (CLL)/prolymphocytic leukemia (PL)/small lymphocytic lymphoma (SLL): CD19+, CD20+, CD79a+, CD5+ (may be negative in PL), CD23+, CD43+, CD11c−/+, CD10−, sIg+ (faint)
- Lymphoplasmacytoid lymphoma: CD19+, CD20+, CD22+, CD79a+, CD5−, CD10−, CD43+/−, sIg+, cIg+ (strong)
- Mantle cell lymphoma: CD19+, CD20+, CD79a+, CD5+, CD23−, CD10−, CD43+, CD11c−, sIg+
- Follicle center cell lymphoma, follicular (follicular small cleaved, mixed and large cell lymphoma in the working formulation): CD19+, CD20+, CD79a+, CD10+/−, CD5−, CD23−/+, CD43−, CD11c−, sIg+
- Marginal zone B-cell lymphoma: CD19+, CD20+, CD22+, CD79a+, CD5−, CD10−, CD23−, CD43−/+, CD11c+/−, sIg+, cIg+ (40%)
- Hairy cell leukemia: CD19+, CD20+, CD22+, CD79a+, CD5−, CD10−, CD23−, CD11c+ (strong), CD25+, FMC7+, CD103+, sIg+
- Plasma cell myeloma: CD19−, CD20−, CD22−, CD79a+/−, CD45−/+, HLA-DR−/+, CD38+, EMA−/+, CD43+/−, CD56+/−, sIg−, cIg+

- Diffuse large B-cell lymphoma: CD19+, CD20+, CD22+, CD79a+, CD45+/−, CD5−/+, CD10−/+, sIg+/−, cIg−/+
- Burkitt's lymphoma: CD19+, CD20+, CD22+, CD79a+, CD10+, CD5−, CD23−, sIg+
- T-cell chronic lymphocytic leukemia (T-CLL): CD7+, CD2+, CD3+, CD5+, CD4+/8− (65%), CD4+/8+ (21%), CD4−/8+ (rare), CD25−
- Large granular lymphocyte (LGL) leukemia (T-cell type): CD2+, CD3+, CD5−, CD7−, TCR+, CD4−, CD8+, CD16+, CD56−, CD57+/−, CD25−
- Large granular lymphocyte (LGL) leukemia (NK-cell type): CD2+, CD3−, TCR−, CD4−, CD8+/−, CD16+, CD56+/−, CD57+/−
- Peripheral T-cell lymphoma: CD3+/−, CD2+/−, CD5+/−, CD7+/−, CD4+/−, CD8+/− (CD4>CD8, may be CD4−/CD8−), CD20− (rare +), CD19−
- Mycosis fungoides/Sézary syndrome (MF/SS): CD2+, CD3+, CD5+, CD7+ (one third), CD4+ (most), CD8+ (rare), CD25−
- Adult T-cell leukemia/lymphoma: CD2+, CD3+, CD5+, CD7−, CD4+, CD25+, CD8+ (rare)

11

MICROBIOLOGY AND VIROLOGY

Appropriate specimen collection and transport are essential for microbiologic testing. A wide variety of special requirements exist because of the fastidiousness of certain microorganisms. The majority of calls from clinicians deal with specimen collection and transport issues. Additionally the pathologist may be called upon by the laboratory to convey certain results to the patient's physician depending on hospital and other regulations.

■ SPECIMEN COLLECTION AND TRANSPORT REQUIREMENTS

These are summarized in Table 11–1. Inappropriately collected and transported specimens should not be processed, and a repeat specimen should be requested.

■ ANAEROBIC CULTURES

Anaerobic cultures should be ordered specifically and are not routinely performed on most specimens. Strict anaerobic conditions are necessary in the collection and transport of specimens for anaerobic cultures. Specimens from sites that normally contain flora are not acceptable.

■ ROUTINE BLOOD CULTURES

The ideal time to collect blood for suspected bacteremia or fungemia is just before a chill. This is usually not possible to identify, and so specimens should be collected immediately after the onset of fever and chills. Three, and often two, separate blood cultures drawn within 24 hours are adequate per septic episode and will show positive results in 99% of patients with intravascular infection. Cultures should be drawn at 30- to 60-minute intervals but can be drawn simultaneously from different sites if antimicrobial therapy needs to be started urgently. Blood should be collected by fresh peripheral venous puncture. Blood from indwelling catheters should not be used except for quantitative blood cultures (discussed later). The volume of blood cultured should be 20 to 30 mL per culture (from multiple sites) to detect low levels of organisms. Lower volumes are acceptable from pediatric patients. A 1 : 10 ratio of blood-to-broth medium volume is considered optimal; however, newer culture systems use higher ratios and can accommodate larger quantities of blood in each bottle. If slow-growing microorganisms are suspected, special culture media can be used, and the specimen can be kept longer than usual. This needs to be indicated to the microbiology laboratory for appropriate handling.

■ BLOOD CULTURES FOR FUNGUS

The lysis-centrifugation system allows greater recovery of fungal organisms and is the preferred detection medium for such cultures in our laboratory. This system contains reagents that inhibit coagulation and the complement cascade and can lyse blood cells. The specimen is centrifuged, and the sediment is then plated on

Text continued on page 166

**Table 11–1 □ SPECIMEN REQUIREMENTS FOR SELECTED
TESTS IN MICROBIOLOGY AND VIROLOGY**

Test	Specimen	Comments
Acid-fast *(Mycobacterium)* culture and smear	See Table 11–4	Swabs are not acceptable
Anaerobic culture	*Suprapubic urine, sterile tissues or fluids, deep wound aspirates:* in anaerobic transport tube	Body sites that normally harbor anaerobic flora are not acceptable Do not refrigerate
Bartonella culture (cat-scratch disease)	*Lymph node or skin biopsy specimen or aspirate:* in sterile container *Blood:* 10-mL (adults), 1.5-mL (pediatric) Isolator tube	
Biopsy culture	*Tissue:* 5–10 mm^3 in sterile container	Specimens in preservative, e.g., formalin, are unacceptable
	Bone marrow: 1.5-mL Isolator tube	Submit multiple pieces if additional cultures are requested
Blood culture for fungus	10-mL Isolator tube	Isolator tubes are used for invasive infections with molds; routine blood culture bottles are sufficient for yeasts
Blood culture for *Mycobacterium*	3–5 mL in special mycobacterial culture (e.g., 13A Bactec) bottle	
Blood culture, quantitative (for suspected line infections)	1.5-mL Isolator tubes from each port (labeled by site); include a peripheral sample at the same time	Clotted or partially filled tubes are unacceptable Line samples without a peripheral sample are unacceptable
Blood culture, routine	8–10 mL (adult), 1–3 mL (pediatric) for aerobic bottles 7–10 mL for anaerobic bottles	Notify lab if *Brucella* spp. or culture-negative endocarditis is suspected

Table continued on following page

Table 11–1 □ **SPECIMEN REQUIREMENTS FOR SELECTED TESTS IN MICROBIOLOGY AND VIROLOGY** *Continued*

Test	Specimen	Comments
Blood smear for parasites	Bedside thick and thin smears (for malaria and babesiosis) Venous blood in EDTA (purple top) (for all parasites)	For suspected malaria, submit at least three specimens within 24 hours
Body fluid culture	1–2 mL in sterile container; dialysis bag effluent	
Bordetella pertussis/ parapertussis by polymerase chain reaction (PCR)	Nasopharyngeal swab	
Chlamydia trachomatis culture	Respiratory, eye, genital swabs or tissues in virus/ *Chlamydia* transport medium Body fluids in sterile container	Transport at 4°C
Clostridium difficile toxin assay	*Stool:* 2 mL in plastic cup	Test performed by enzyme immunoassay Rectal swabs or stool in viral transport medium is unacceptable
Cytomegalovirus (CMV) antigenemia assay	*Blood:* 8 mL in heparin (green top) tube	Test performed by fluorescent antibody stain Results reported as number of positive cells/50,000 WBC; values considered high risk for disease are: >1 for allogeneic bone marrow transplantation (BMT) >5 for autologous BMT >10 for renal transplant recipient Rapidly rising levels for any patient

Table 11–1 □ SPECIMEN REQUIREMENTS FOR SELECTED TESTS IN MICROBIOLOGY AND VIROLOGY *Continued*

Test	Specimen	Comments
DNA probe *(Neisseria gonorrhoeae/ Chlamydia trachomatis)*	*Cervical, urethral, eye:* commercial swab transport kits	Test performed by nonamplified nucleic acid hybridization
Eye or ear culture	Swab	
Foreign body culture	Submit in sterile container	
Fungus culture	*Tissue:* 5–10 mm^3 *Bone marrow:* 1.5-mL Isolator tube *Hair, nails, skin:* sterile dry container *Fluid or aspirate:* at least 3–5 mL in sterile container *Urine:* at least 10 mL in sterile container	
Fungus culture (yeast only)	*Stool, vaginal, mouth, throat:* swab	Recommended when screening for *Candida* spp.
Genital culture	*Urethral, vaginal, cervical, amniotic fluid, endometrium, prostatic fluid, ovarian tissue, testicular tissue:* swab or fluid/ aspirate (2–3 mL in sterile container)	Dry swabs are unacceptable
Group B streptococci screen	1 or 2 swabs of vaginal introitus and anorectum	Recommended for all pregnant women
Herpes simplex virus (HSV) PCR	*Cerebrospinal fluid:* >0.2 mL in sterile container	
HIV quantitative PCR	*Whole blood:* 5–10 mL in EDTA (purple top) *EDTA plasma:* in sterile polypropylene tube	Blood must reach lab within 5 hours of collection Plasma must be separated within 6 hours of specimen collection

Table continued on following page

Table 11–1 □ **SPECIMEN REQUIREMENTS FOR SELECTED TESTS IN MICROBIOLOGY AND VIROLOGY** *Continued*

Test	Specimen	Comments
Human papillomavirus detection/typing	*Cervical swab, small anogenital biopsy:* commercial collection and transport kit *Large anogenital biopsy:* use sterile container *Cervical broom:* use preservative solution for Thin-Prep pap smears	Swab in transport medium: 4°C Biopsy specimen in transport medium: 4°C or room temperature Cervical broom in solution: room temperature
Influenza A antigen	Nasal wash or aspirate in specimen trap	Sensitivity on adult patients is ~50%
Intestinal culture	*Stool:* 1–2 g in plastic container *Bile:* 1–2 mL in sterile container Rectal swab	Contaminated specimens are unacceptable Transport within 1 hour Routine cultures include *Salmonella, Shigella, Campylobacter,* staphylococci, *Aeromonas, Plesiomonas, E. coli* O157:H7
Legionella culture or direct fluorescent antibody stain	*Sputum, BAL fluid:* 2–3 mL in sterile cup *Tissue:* 5–10 mm³	Transport within 1 hour Refrigerate if delayed Do not add saline to specimen
Legionella urine antigen	*Urine:* in sterile container	Test performed by enzyme immunoassay Positive results are presumptive evidence of infection with *Legionella pneumophila* serogroup 1

Table 11–1 □ **SPECIMEN REQUIREMENTS FOR SELECTED TESTS IN MICROBIOLOGY AND VIROLOGY** *Continued*

Test	Specimen	Comments
Mycoplasma culture (genital)	*Cervical, vaginal, urethral swabs:* in genital *Mycoplasma* transport medium *Urine, semen, prostatic fluid:* in sterile container *Respiratory secretions* (if <1 year of age)	Transport at 4°C unless in genital *Mycoplasma* transport medium (which can be left at room temperature)
Mycoplasma culture (respiratory)	*Respiratory, CSF, synovial fluid specimens:* swabs or tissues in *Mycoplasma pneumoniae* transport medium, body fluids in sterile container	Transport at 4°C unless in *Mycoplasma pneumoniae* transport medium (which can be left at room temperature)
Neisseria screen culture	*Cervical, vaginal (prepubescent females), urethral, throat, rectum, eye:* swab *Martin-Lewis plates:* inoculated at bedside	Dry swabs, old or dry plates are unacceptable Transport immediately
Parasites	*Urine, sputum, tissue:* in clean container	
Parasites, stool (ova and parasites)	*Stool:* in collection vial with fixative or in clean container	
Pneumocystis fluorescent antibody stain	*Induced sputum:* >0.5 mL *Bronchial wash, BAL, endotracheal aspirate, pleural fluid, lung biopsy:* in sterile container	Expectorated sputum is unacceptable
Respiratory culture, quantitative	*BAL:* 13 mL in sterile container *Bronchial brush:* in sterile transport vials	Significance of culture growth is assessed by colony count

Table continued on following page

Table 11–1 □ **SPECIMEN REQUIREMENTS FOR SELECTED TESTS IN MICROBIOLOGY AND VIROLOGY** *Continued*

Test	Specimen	Comments
Respiratory culture, routine	*Throat:* swab *Nasopharyngeal:* minitipped swab *Sputum, bronchial washings, endotracheal aspirates:* 3–5 mL in sterile container	
Respiratory syncytial virus (RSV) antigen	Nasal wash or aspirate in specimen trap	Test performed by enzyme immunoassay Transport at 4°C
Rotavirus antigen	*Stool:* 1 g in plastic cup	Test performed by enzyme immunoassay
Treponema pallidum fluorescent antibody stain	Lesion exudate on glass slides	Air dry slides without fixatives
Urine culture	1 mL in sterile container	Specify type of urine for correct culture work-up and interpretation
Vaginitis, bacterial	Vaginal swab	
Vaginitis, *Trichomonas*	*Urethral/vaginal secretions:* swab	Transport immediately
Vaginitis, yeast	Vaginal swab	
Viral culture, general	*Swabs or tissues:* in viral transport medium *Body fluids or feces:* in sterile container	Transport at 4°C
Wound culture	Aspirates (rather than swabs) in sterile container	Avoid contact with skin surface

agar. This allows better recovery of fungi, *Staphylococcus aureus*, and some Enterobacteriaceae and can be used for quantitative cultures as well (discussed below). However, it is very labor intensive.

■ QUANTITATIVE BLOOD CULTURES

Quantitative blood cultures are useful for establishing intravascular catheters as a source of infection. Blood is collected from each catheter (and each lumen of a multilumen catheter), and at the same time, one or more peripheral blood cultures are drawn. A specified amount of blood should be collected from each site and the lysis-centrifugation system can be used for this purpose. The colony counts from the catheter sites and the peripheral blood are quantitated, and if the catheter count is five times greater than the peripheral count, the catheter site is implicated as the source of infection and is an indication for changing the catheter. To obtain accurate results, however, all sites must be sampled at the same time, and the tubes should be filled completely (thereby ensuring that an equal amount of blood is collected from each site).

■ BLOOD CULTURES FOR DETECTION OF VIRUSES

A few viruses can be detected in the blood. Viremia is a transient part of several viral infections, but in some cases it is the predominant site of involvement in pathogenesis. Specimen requirements are summarized in Table 11–2. Some of these tests are performed by ref-

Table 11–2 □ SPECIMEN REQUIREMENTS FOR OPTIMAL DETECTION OF VIRUSES FOUND IN BLOOD

Virus	Blood Specimen Requirements		
	Type Collected	Fraction Used for Detection	Volume (mL)
Cytomegalovirus	With anticoagulant*	Leukocytes	5–10
Enteroviruses	With or without anticoagulant*	Serum or leukocytes	5–10
Human immuno-deficiency virus	Heparinized	Mononuclear cells or plasma	10†
Human herpesvirus–6	Heparinized	Mononuclear cells	5–10
Parvovirus B19	Without anti-coagulant	Serum	5–10
Arthropod-borne viruses‡	With or without anticoagulant	Leukocytes or homogenized clot	5–10

From Henry JB: Clinical Diagnosis and Management by Laboratory Methods, 19th ed. Philadelphia, WB Saunders Co, 1996, p 1316.

*Heparin or EDTA may be used for cytomegalovirus; heparin, citrate, or EDTA for enteroviruses.

†Smaller volumes are acceptable from infants.

‡Includes viruses of eastern, western, and Venezuelan equine encephalitis; St. Louis and California encephalitis; yellow fever; dengue; and Colorado tick fever.

erence laboratories only. If cytomegalovirus is suspected, a cytospin preparation of leukocytes can be stained with monoclonal antibodies to detect viremia and provides a more rapid result than culture does.

■ BLOOD FOR DETECTION OF PARASITES

Blood should be collected in anticoagulant and transported to the laboratory at once. Different types of smears can be made to visualize different parasitic organisms. Thin smears are made for hematologic examinations and stained with Giemsa stain. They are useful for identifying the species of *Plasmodium, Babesia, Trypanosoma, Ehrlichia,* and microfilariae. One prepares thick smears by placing a drop of blood on a slide and spreading it with another slide to cover an area of 1 square centimeter. It is stained with Giemsa stain without fixation and is useful for detecting all parasites. One prepares direct mounts by placing a drop of blood on a slide, covering it with a coverslip, and examining it under a microscope. This is useful for detecting microfilariae and the trypomastigotes of trypanosomiasis.

■ CEREBROSPINAL FLUID CULTURES

Many different microbiologic agents can cause meningitis, and cerebrospinal fluid (CSF) is an ideal specimen for diagnosis of such infections. Bacterial causes of meningitis are summarized in Table 11–3. Usually CSF is collected by lumbar puncture, and three to four tubes are submitted to the laboratory. The first tube should be used for a cell count and differential, the second tube for Gram stain and microbiologic cultures, and the third and fourth tubes for protein, glucose, and other tests including serology and cytology. Specimens should be processed immediately. They can be held at room temperature for a brief interval; if viral cultures are requested, a portion of the specimens should be refrigerated.

■ CSF ANTIGEN SCREEN IN CSF

Latex agglutination tests are available for detecting antigens of group B streptococci, *Streptococcus pneumoniae,* some serotypes of *Neisseria meningitidis, Escherichia coli,* and *Haemophilus influenzae.* These tests can be performed on the supernatant of a centrifuged specimen, the filtrate of a filtered specimen, or the original specimen. Their sensitivity, however, is not significantly greater than that of a simple Gram stain, and because they are much more expensive to perform, their routine use should be discouraged. Their main role is in confirming a Gram-stain result or in cases of partially treated meningitis.

Table 11–3 □ COMMON BACTERIAL CAUSES OF ACUTE MENINGITIS BY AGE

Age	Organisms
Neonates—3 months	Group B streptococci
	Escherichia coli
	*Listeria monocytogenes**
	Streptococcus pneumoniae
4 months—6 years	*Haemophilus influenzae,* type b†
6 years—45 years	*Neisseria meningitidis*
>45 years	*Streptococcus pneumoniae*
	Listeria monocytogenes
	Group B streptococci

From Henry JB: Clinical Diagnosis and Management by Laboratory Methods, 19th ed. Philadelphia, WB Saunders Co, 1996, p 1317.
*May cause meningitis in immunocompromised individuals in all age groups.
†Incidence has declined as a result of vaccination.

■ DETECTION OF *CRYPTOCOCCUS NEOFORMANS* IN CSF

Several rapid methods are available for detection of *Cryptococcus neoformans* in cerebrospinal fluid. One can make an India ink stain by mixing one drop of CSF with one drop of India ink on a slide and looking for encapsulated yeast cells of *Cryptococcus neoformans* under high power. This test has a low sensitivity except in HIV-infected persons. Either the cryptococcal latex agglutination test or the enzyme-linked immunosorbent assay has sensitivities over 90% and also is highly specific. These two tests can be performed on the supernatant of a centrifuged specimen or the filtrate of a filtered specimen, in addition to the original specimen itself. The latex agglutination test can be performed easily and does not require any special equipment. It should be done before culture or on a separate specimen. Positive and negative controls are included with the test kit. Equivocal results can be repeated when a 1:1 dilution of the specimen is used.

■ RESPIRATORY SPECIMENS

Nasopharyngeal specimens are useful in detecting viral infections, diphtheria, pertussis, and *Chlamydia trachomatis* pneumonia in infants. Nasopharyngeal aspirates and washings are better than swabs for culture. Throat swabs are collected most often to diagnose group A streptococcal pharyngitis but can also be useful in detecting agents of acute epiglottitis, gonorrhea, viruses shed in oral secretions, diphtheria, Vincent's angina, and *Mycoplasma pneumoniae* pneumonia. Rapid tests are available for identifying group A streptococcus in throat swabs. Two swabs should be collected; the rapid test should be performed on the first swab, and the second swab should be used for culture if the rapid test is negative because the sensitivity of the rapid test is low. Sputum specimens are used for the etiologic diagnosis of pneumonia. Specimens should be evaluated for contamination by saliva with a Gram stain. The presence of more than 10 epithelial cells per low-power field is considered significant contamination, and such specimens should be rejected. However, if the suspected etiologic agent is *Mycoplasma pneumoniae*, mycobacteria, or *Legionella* species, or if the specimen is induced sputum, screening is not required.

■ DETECTION OF *PNEUMOCYSTIS CARINII*

Bronchoalveolar lavage specimens are preferable to sputum for detection of *Pneumocystis carinii*. The yield of sputum specimens is particularly low in patients with underlying diseases other than HIV. Several different stains, such as silver stains, calcofluor white, and toluidine blue, can be used to visualize the cysts. The cysts are 5 μm in diameter and round or collapsed ("helmet" shaped). Giemsa stains can demonstrate the sporozoites, which are much smaller and more difficult than the others to visualize. Immunofluorescence techniques using monoclonal antibodies are now available and are more sensitive and specific than conventional stains. In our laboratory, the immunofluorescent stain is performed on a *stat.* basis on bronchoalveolar lavage specimens if *Pneumocystis carinii* is suspected. Conventional stains are used if specimens are also received for cytologic or histologic examination.

■ DETECTION OF MYCOBACTERIA

Common specimens obtained for isolation of mycobacteria are listed in Table 11–4. Specimens from sites that normally have microbial colonization should be decontaminated before processing, whereas those from sterile sites can be processed directly. The sensitivity of smear and culture can be increased further when the specimen is concentrated after decontamination. Specimens are processed for acid-fast stains and culture. Broth and solid media are available for culture; the former allow a faster turnaround time for detection of growth than the latter. Definite identification is based on colony morphology and biochemical tests; more recently the use of DNA probes and analysis of long-chain fatty acids by gas-liquid chromatography or high-performance liquid chromatography has enabled rapid identification.

Table 11–4 □ DISEASES CAUSED BY MYCOBACTERIA AND SPECIMENS FOR DIAGNOSIS

Disease	Mycobacterium Species*	Specimens
Pulmonary	tuberculosis, kansasii, MAC, xenopi, szulgai, malmoense, simiae	Sputum (early morning, deep cough, on 3 consecutive days), BAL, gastric contents, lung tissue, pleural fluid
Disseminated	tuberculosis, MAC	Blood, bone marrow, involved tissue
Lymphadenitis	tuberculosis, MAC, scrofulaceum	Lymph node aspirate or biopsy
Skin, soft tissue	ulcerans, fortuitum-chelonae, marinum, haemophilum leprae	Aspirate or biopsy of lesions (swabs should be discouraged) Smears of nasal secretions and skin slits, biopsy of lesion
Musculoskeletal	tuberculosis, fortuitum-chelonei, marinum	Joint fluid, synovium, bone
Nervous system	tuberculosis leprae	CSF, brain tissue Peripheral nerve biopsy
Genitourinary	tuberculosis	Urine (early morning–voided specimen on 3 consecutive days), involved tissue—kidney, endometrium, fallopian tubes, prostate, seminal vesicles, epididymis
Gastrointestinal	tuberculosis, MAC	Tissue, feces
Peritonitis	tuberculosis	Peritoneal biopsy, peritoneal fluid
Hepatitis	tuberculosis, MAC	Liver tissue
Pericarditis	tuberculosis	Pericardium, pericardial fluid

Modified from Woods GL: Mycobacteria. *In* Woods GL, Gutierrez Y: Diagnostic Pathology of Infectious Diseases. Philadelphia, Lea & Febiger, 1993, p 378.

*Species listed are potential pathogens most commonly involved.

MAC = *M. avium-intracellulare* complex; BAL = bronchoalveolar lavage; CSF = cerebrospinal fluid.

■ ACID-FAST STAINS

The laboratory is often required to urgently perform an acid-fast stain on specimens from patients with suspected mycobacterial disease. Two types of stains are used for detecting acid-fast organisms—the fluorochrome stains (auramine-rhodamine, or auramine-O) and the carbol-fuchsin stains (Ziehl-Neelsen or Kinyoun's). Although the specificity of these stains is excellent (99%), the sensitivity is variable (25–75%, higher with fluorochrome stains). Therefore clinicians should not use a negative result as the sole basis for discontinuing respiratory isolation. Acid-fast stains can also be used to monitor therapy in patients who were initially smear positive. Fluorochrome-stained smears can be examined at lower magnification than smears stained with carbol-fuchsin, and therefore a larger area can be screened in less time. Positive fluorochrome stains are usually confirmed by a carbol-fuchsin stain because the latter stains only viable organisms and allows better visualization of the morphology of the organisms than the other type does. If stains are performed on an unconcentrated specimen, this should be indicated in the report because it may decrease sensitivity. General guidelines for performing and interpreting the two stains are as follows:

Kinyoun's (cold) carbol-fuchsin stain:

- Heat fix the smear.
- Cover with carbol-fuchsin stain for 5 minutes.
- Rinse with water.
- Decolorize with acid-alcohol for 2 minutes or until no more stain appears in the washing.
- Counterstain with methylene blue for 1–2 minutes.
- Rinse with water and dry.
- Examine 300 fields under 100× oil-immersion objective. Mycobacteria are purple to red, slightly curved rods (1 to 10 μm long and 0.2 to 0.6 μm wide). Report as outlined in Table 11–5.

Auramine-fluorochrome stain:

- Heat fix the smear.
- Cover with auramine for 15 minutes.
- Rinse with water.
- Decolorize with acid-alcohol for 2 minutes.
- Rinse with water.
- Flood smear with potassium permanganate for 2–4 minutes.
- Rinse with water and dry.
- Examine 100 fields under 25× objective on a fluorescent microscope. Mycobacteria show bright yellow fluorescence against a black background. Report as outlined in Table 11–5.

NOTE: For both techniques, the recommended area of the smear to be examined is three sweeps along the long axis of the slide; this

Table 11–5 □ **GUIDELINES FOR REPORTING SMEARS FOR ACID-FAST BACILLI**

AFB with Carbol-Fuchsin Stain (1000×) (No.)	AFB with Fluorochrome Stain (450×) (No.)	Report
0	0	No AFB seen
1–2/300 F (3 sweeps)	1–2/70 F (1½ sweeps)	Doubtful; repeat
1–9/100 F	2–18/50 F (1 sweep)	1+
1–9/10 F	4–36/10 F	2+
1–9 F	4–36 F	3+
>9 F	>36 F	4+

Modified from Kent PT, Kubica GP: Public Health Mycobacteriology: A Guide for the Level III Laboratory. Atlanta, US Department of Health and Human Services, 1985.
AFB = acid-fast bacilli; sweep = scanning full length of a smear; F = field.

corresponds roughly to 300 fields using the 100× objective and 100 fields using the 25× objective. Appropriate positive and negative control slides should be stained and examined along with the patient's smear.

Cultures are required for identification of mycobacterial species. Rapid methods, including the polymerase chain reaction (PCR), may be applied to smear-positive specimens for early diagnosis.

■ GENITAL SPECIMENS

Specimens for detection of *Neisseria gonorrhoeae* should be inoculated directly on a selective medium such as modified Thayer-Martin medium and placed in a container with a CO_2-generating tablet. These specimens should be transported at room temperature and should never be refrigerated. *Chlamydia trachomatis* can be detected by culture using special culture media or by direct fluorescent antibody staining. Also available are enzyme immunoassays and DNA probes, which have specific collection media included in the manufacturer's kit.

Viruses are optimally detected by culture. Viral cytopathic effect can be seen on smear preparations from visible lesions (Tzanck smear). Both air-dried (Wright-Giemsa or Diff-Quik stained) and 95% alcohol-fixed (Papanicolaou- or hematoxylin and eosin-stained) smears should be made for best results. The diagnosis of syphilis is based largely on serologic tests, but dark-field examination of exudate from skin lesions may show spirochetes as tight coils with pointed ends.

■ FECAL SPECIMENS

Stool is the preferred specimen for isolating adenoviruses, enteroviruses, and the viruses responsible for gastroenteritis. If specific bacterial pathogens are sought, the laboratory should be informed. For example, isolation of *Yersinia enterocolitica* requires incubation at room temperature. Isolation of *Clostridium* species requires strict anaerobic conditions. Pseudomembranous colitis associated with *Clostridium difficile* toxin is best diagnosed by cell culture assay for cytotoxin. Stool should be processed within 2 hours of collection or stored in the refrigerator. Diagnosis of ova and parasites in stool may require more than one specimen. Although 90% of all infections are diagnosed on the first specimen, up to three specimens may be required to detect some parasites such as amoebas. Special stains are required for some organisms including *Cryptosporidium*, Microsporida, and *Cyclospora*.

■ REPORTING OF RESULTS

Communicable diseases need to be reported to local authorities. A list of diseases and reporting requirements for New York State is listed in Table 11–6. Public health authorities have different protocols for reporting, and phoned or faxed reports may be required for certain diseases in addition to mailed copies. Laboratory personnel are usually well aware of such regulations, but it is useful to have a list readily available for review. It is essential that such public health requirements be met, both for legal reasons and epidemiologic concerns.

The laboratory is also required to report certain results to the Centers for Disease Control and Prevention (CDC). In addition, most laboratories have their own protocols for calling certain results to physicians directly to optimize patient care. Some such results include positive cultures from any site that is usually sterile (such as blood or CSF), positive acid-fast stains or mycobacterial cultures, and positive fungal cultures. It is also important to inform the clinician of the significance of the results, particularly when the results are suggestive of contaminants rather than true pathogens. This helps to prevent unnecessary antimicrobial treatment.

■ SUSCEPTIBILITY TESTING

Most routine bacterial isolates are tested for susceptibility to antimicrobial agents. The choice of drugs tested depends on the organism isolated, local resistance patterns, and patterns of antibiotic use. In many laboratories, a cascade system is used where several drugs are tested, but only a few commonly used drugs are reported; if the

Text continued on page 178

**Table 11–6 □ NEW YORK STATE DEPARTMENT OF HEALTH
REQUIREMENTS FOR REPORTING OF COMMUNICABLE DISEASES**

Agent	Disease	What to Report
Arboviruses: California sero-group virus (La Crosse, James-town, Canyon, etc.), eastern or western equine encephalitis, St. Louis encephali-tis, Powassan en-cephalitis	Viral encephalitis	Positive viral culture, PCR, or serologic evidence for any of the arboviruses
Babesia microti	Babesiosis	Positive blood smear or serologic evidence
*Bacillus anthracis**	Anthrax	Positive culture or IFA
Bordetella pertussis	Pertussis	Positive culture, PCR, or DFA
Borrelia burgdorferi	Lyme disease	Positive culture or serologic evidence
Brucella sp.	Brucellosis	Positive culture, IFA, or serologic evidence
Calymmatobacterium granulomatis	Granuloma inguinale disease	Positive culture
Campylobacter spp.	Campylobacteriosis	Positive culture
Chlamydia psittaci	Psittacosis	Positive culture or serologic evidence
*Clostridium botulinum**	Botulism	Positive culture or toxin in blood or stool
Clostridium tetani	Tetanus	Positive culture
*Corynebacterium diphtheriae**	Diphtheria	Positive culture from throat, skin, or histopathology
Cryptosporidium parvum	Cryptosporidiosis	Positive oocyst or antigen noted by any method
Cyclospora cayetanensis	Cyclosporiasis	Positive oocyst in stool noted by any method
Ehrlichia sp.	Ehrlichiosis	Positive serology, PCR, or culture

*Results have to be communicated immediately by telephone or fax.

AFB = Acid-fast bacillus; DFA = direct fluorescent antibody; IFA = indirect fluorescent antibody; MIC = minimal inhibitory concentration; PCR = polymerase chain reaction.

Table continued on following page

Table 11–6 □ NEW YORK STATE DEPARTMENT OF HEALTH
REQUIREMENTS FOR REPORTING OF COMMUNICABLE
DISEASES *Continued*

Agent	Disease	What to Report
Entamoeba histolytica	Amebiasis	Positive cyst, trophozoite, or antigen noted by any method
Escherichia coli O157:H7	*E. coli* O157 infection	Positive *E. coli* O157 culture from stool
*Francisella tularensis**	Tularemia	Positive culture or significant titer
Giardia duodenalis (lamblia)	Giardiasis	Positive cyst, trophozoite, or antigen by any method
Haemophilus ducreyi	Chancroid	Positive culture or PCR
Haemophilus influenzae	*Haemophilus influenzae* disease (invasive)	Positive culture from otherwise sterile sites such as blood, CSF
Hantavirus	Hantavirus pulmonary syndrome	Positive Hanta IgM or rising IgG serology titer or positive RNA by PCR or positive immunohistochemistry
Hepatitis A virus	Hepatitis A	Positive serology result for IgM anti-HAV
Hepatitis B virus	Hepatitis B	Positive serology result for HBsAg confirmed by neutralization or IgM anti-HBc
Hepatitis C virus	Hepatitis C	All positive confirmatory tests
Histoplasma capsulatum	Histoplasmosis	Positive culture or serologic evidence
Legionella spp.	Legionellosis	Positive culture, nucleic acid, DFA, or urinary antigen or acute/convalescent serology titer showing a fourfold rise to *L. pneumophila*

Table 11–6 □ **NEW YORK STATE DEPARTMENT OF HEALTH
REQUIREMENTS FOR REPORTING OF COMMUNICABLE
DISEASES** *Continued*

Agent	Disease	What to Report
Measles virus*	Measles	Paired sera showing rising IgG titer, single serum showing measles IgM antibody, or positive viral culture
Mumps virus	Mumps	Paired sera showing rising IgG titer, single serum showing mumps IgM antibody, or positive viral culture
Mycobacterium leprae	Hansen's disease (leprosy)	Positive AFB smear (skin or dermal nerve)
Mycobacterium tuberculosis and *M. bovis**	Tuberculosis	Positive AFB smear, positive culture for *M. tuberculosis* or *M. bovis* from any site, susceptibility test results, or histologic evidence of disease
Neisseria gonorrhoeae	Gonorrhea	Positive by any method
*Neisseria meningitidis**	Meningococcal disease (meningitis)	Positive culture from blood or CSF or Gram stain showing Gram-negative diplococci in CSF or blood
Plasmodium spp.	Malaria	Positive blood smear
Polio virus*	Poliomyelitis	Positive viral culture or PCR
Rabies virus*	Rabies	Results from specialized laboratory
Rickettsia rickettsii	Rocky Mountain spotted fever	Positive culture or serologic evidence or PCR or IFA of lesion or tissue
Rubella virus*	Rubella (German measles)	Paired sera showing rising IgG titer, single serum showing rubella IgM antibody, or positive viral culture

Table continued on following page

Table 11–6 □ NEW YORK STATE DEPARTMENT OF HEALTH
REQUIREMENTS FOR REPORTING OF COMMUNICABLE
DISEASES *Continued*

Agent	Disease	What to Report
Salmonella spp.	Salmonellosis	Positive culture
*Salmonella typhi**	Typhoid fever	Positive culture
Shigella spp.	Shigellosis	Positive culture
*Staphylococcus aureus**	Vancomycin-resistant staphylococcal (VRSA) infection	Isolate showing reduced suscep- tibility to van- comycin
Streptococcus agalactiae (Group B Strep)	Group B streptococcal invasive disease	Positive culture from blood or CSF
*Streptococcus pneumoniae**	Drug-resistant *Streptococcus pneumoniae* inva- sive disease	Antibiotic resistant strains (MIC >0.06 μg/mL for penicillin) from blood or CSF
Streptococcus pyogenes (Group A beta-hemolytic Strep)	Group A streptococcal invasive disease	Positive culture from sterile sites such as blood, CSF, or any site from a patient with necrotizing fasciitis
*Treponema pallidum**	Syphilis	Any positive serology or dark-field mi- croscopy result showing trepo- nemes or DFA
Trichinella sp.	Trichinosis	Positive biopsy or serology result
Vibrio cholerae: O1 or O139*	Cholera	Positive culture or significant serology result
Vibrio non O1 spp.	Vibriosis	Positive culture
Yellow fever virus	Yellow fever	Positive culture or significant serology result
Yersinia enterocolitica	Yersiniosis	Positive culture
*Yersinia pestis**	Plague	Positive culture or serology result

organism is resistant to those drugs, additional ones are reported as necessary. This helps to curb overuse of newer drugs and delays de- velopment of resistance. A general guideline is presented in Table 11–7; individualized protocols are formulated in conjunction with the infectious disease physicians. Susceptibility testing for my- cobacteria and fungi is less well defined. Standard protocols are available for testing isolates of *Mycobacterium tuberculosis.*

■ SERUM ANTIMICROBIAL ACTIVITY (SCHLICHTER TEST)

The serum killing power assay, or Schlichter test, is an *in vitro* measurement of the antibacterial activity of serum containing antimicrobial agents. Theoretically it is the best measure of the utility of an antimicrobial agent. Serum samples are collected as peak (preferred) or trough specimens, and the bactericidal activity of serial dilutions is assayed. A bactericidal titer of 1:64 (peak) or 1:32 (trough) is predictive of bacteriologic cure. However, failure to achieve these titers does not allow prediction of bacteriologic failure. This test is time consuming and should be used only for refractory infections such as gram-negative sepsis, streptococcal endocarditis, and osteomyelitis. It can be used with measurement of serum drug levels in monitoring therapy.

■ PULMONARY MICROORGANISM SEARCH IN IMMUNOCOMPROMISED PATIENTS

Immunocompromised patients with pulmonary infiltrates or suspected pulmonary infections routinely undergo bronchoscopy to obtain appropriate specimens to search for a variety of microorganisms and, in some instances, to rule out a neoplasm. At our institution, a standard protocol has been established to optimally process such specimens and produce expeditious results. Both bronchoalveolar lavage and transbronchial biopsy specimens are obtained and processed as follows:

Bronchoalveolar Lavage

Separate specimens are submitted for:

- *Cytopathology*
  Cytologic evaluation
  Cell counts
  Silver stain (for fungus and *Pneumocystis carinii*)
- *Microbiology*
  Gram stain
  Routine culture and sensitivity
  Acid-fast stain and culture
  Fungus culture
  Legionella culture and direct fluorescent antibody stain for *Legionella*
- *Virology*
  Viral cultures (use viral transport medium)
  Chlamydia cultures (use *Chlamydia* transport medium)

Table 11–7 □ GUIDELINES FOR SELECTION OF ANTIBACTERIAL AGENTS FOR SUSCEPTIBILITY TESTING*

	Staphylococci	Enterococci	Nonenterococcal Streptococci	Pseudomonas	Enterobacteriaceae
Amikacin				P	P
Ampicillin	S	P			P
Ampicillin/sulbactam (or amoxicillin/clavulanate)	S				S
Azlocillin (or mezlocillin or piperacillin or ticarcillin)				P	
Aztreonam				S	S
Cefamandole (or cefonicid or cefuroxime)					S
Cefotaxime (or cefoperazone or ceftazidime or ceftizoxime or ceftriaxone or moxalactam)					P
Cefoxitin (or cefotetan)					S
Ceftazidime (or cefoperazone)				P	
Cephalothin	P		P		P†
Chloramphenicol	S			S	S
Ciprofloxacin	S		P	S	S
Clindamycin	P				
Erythromycin	P	U	P		
Gentamicin (or tobramycin)	S	S§		P	P

Agent				
Imipenem		S		S
Mezlocillin (or piperacillin or ticarcillin)				P
Netilmicin		S		S
Oxacillin (or methicillin or nafcillin)				
Penicillin G	P‡			S, U
Tetracycline	P			S
Ticarcillin/clavulanate	S			P
Trimethoprim/sulfamethoxazole	P	S	S¶	
Vancomycin			S	
Cinoxacin (or nalidixic acid)	U	U		U
Nitrofurantoin	U	U		U
Norfloxacin	U		U	U
Trimethoprim	U			U

From Woods GL, Washington SA: In vitro testing of antimicrobial agents. *In* Henry JB: Clinical Diagnosis and Management by Laboratory Methods, 19th ed. Philadelphia, WB Saunders Co, 1996, p 1172.

*P = Primary agents to be tested routinely; S = secondary agents to be tested under special circumstances, such as in institutions harboring endemic or epidemic resistance to one or more of the primary agents, for therapy of patients allergic to a primary agent, or as an epidemiologic aid; U = urinary tract–specific agent to be tested against urinary isolates only.

†Although cephalothin can be used to predict the *in vitro* activity of other first-generation cephalosporins, cefazolin should not be used for the same purpose because cefazolin is more active than other first-generation cephalosporins versus *E. coli.*

‡Oxacillin- (or methicillin- or nafcillin–) resistant staphylococci should be considered resistant to cephalosporins, penicillins (including combinations with β-lactamase inhibitors), and imipenem.

§Gentamicin and streptomycin should be tested at a concentration of 500 or 2000 µg/mL and 2000 µg/ml, respectively, to detect high-level resistant strains that are not synergistically affected by the combination of a penicillin and a respective aminoglycoside.

¶Applies only to species other than *P. aeruginosa.*

- *Mycoplasma* cultures (use *Mycoplasma pneumoniae* transport medium)

Transbronchial Biopsy

Separate specimens are submitted for:

- *Surgical pathology.* Apart from routine H&E sections, special stains for acid-fast organisms, fungi, and *Pneumocystis carinii* can be ordered. Transbronchial biopsy specimens can be rush processed on 2- to 4-hour processor cycles to avoid delays.
- *Microbiology*
  Gram stain
  Routine culture and sensitivity
  Anaerobic culture
  Legionella culture and direct fluorescent antibody stain for *Legionella*
  Acid-fast stain and culture
  Fungus culture

Procuring appropriate specimens for culture at the outset is essential for meaningful microbiologic results. The clinician and pathologist should consider all possibilities so as not to miss unusual pathogens. The role of the pathologist is most often to help determine the best specimen collection and handling option. With increasing use of rapid identification techniques (immunofluorescent probes, DNA probes, PCR, etc.) the role of the microbiology laboratory will expand, and these modalities will become available on a *stat.* basis, in addition to traditional screening tests such as the Gram stain.

CHEMISTRY AND IMMUNOLOGY

Interpretation of chemistry and immunology results is of foremost importance. Pathologists on call are also involved in specimen collection and handling, resolving questions about suspect results (see Chapter 4), clarifying and translating results with additional or confirmatory testing, and calling out significantly abnormal results to physicians or other appropriate persons when laboratory personnel are unable to accomplish such duties.

■ CRITICALLY ABNORMAL RESULTS

So-called panic values are abnormal test results that go beyond certain predetermined limits and indicate pronounced physiologic alterations. Such results need to be communicated immediately to the patient's physician, and such communication is usually done by the technologist for patients in the hospital. Critically abnormal results on specimens from outpatients are sometimes more difficult to communicate because the patient's physician may not be available. Most clinics have physicians on call who can be informed of the abnormal results and who will then try to contact the patient. It is important to remember that inappropriate specimen collection and handling can contribute to critically abnormal results, and one should keep this in mind, particularly when analyzing outpatient specimens (since these specimens are from patients who are probably not critically ill). A list of critically abnormal results in chemistry used by our laboratory is presented in Table 12–1. It is also appropriate to initiate a confirmation request when there is any doubt about validity of determination (Chapter 4).

Table 12–1 □ PROCEDURE FOR CRITICALLY ABNORMAL RESULTS (PANIC-VALUES) IN CHEMISTRY

The chemistry values that must be called immediately by the technologist to the physician or charge nurse in the requesting unit are as follows:
 1. Acetaminophen >50 μg/mL
 2. Bicarbonate (CO_2) <10 or >40 mmol/L
 3. Blood gases: pH <7.25, >7.50; Po_2 <50 mm Hg; Pco_2 <20, >70
 4. Calcium <2.5 or >5.9 mEq/L
 5. Carbamazepine >12 μg/mL
 6. Cortisol <5 or >50 μg/dL
 7. Digoxin >3.0 ng/mL
 8. Ethosuximide >100 μg/mL
 9. Glucose <50 or >500 mg/dL
10. Lead, blood >25 μg/dL
11. Lidocaine >10 μg/mL
12. Lithium >1.2 mmol/L
13. Phenobarbital >50 μg/mL
14. Phenytoin >30 μg/mL
15. Potassium <3.0 or >5.9 mmol/L
16. Primidone >12 μg/mL
17. Procainamide and NAPA (total) >30 μg/mL
18. Quinidine >10 μg/mL
19. Salicylate >50 mg/dL
20. Sodium <120 or >160 mmol/L
21. Theophylline >30 μg/mL
22. Thiocyanate >12 mg/dL
23. Thyroxine >30 ng/dL
24. Valproic acid >100 μg/mL
25. Vancomycin >30 μg/mL
26. Urine protein greater than 4 g per 24-hour urine collection

If every effort made to contact a physician or nurse caring for the patient fails, the Clinical Pathology resident assigned to chemistry should be advised and should contact clinical house staff or attending as required. The Clinical Chemistry resident is also responsible for confirming and reporting immediately any monoclonal bands on serum protein electrophoresis.

■ SPECIMEN REQUIREMENTS

Most determinations in chemistry are performed on serum though plasma is also used and may have advantages in selected testing. Table 12–2 lists specimen requirements for common determinations in chemistry and immunology. Tubes for blood collection are color coded depending on the nature of anticoagulant used (Table 12–3).

■ DRUG INTERACTIONS

Abnormal test results may be the result of drug interactions. Drugs can interfere with assays either *in vivo* (physiologic interference) or *in vitro* (physical or chemical interference). An extensive list of drug interactions is available (Table 12–4) and should be a ready reference for evaluation of suspected interferences.

■ CHEMISTRY MEASUREMENTS

Salient features of selected chemistry measurements that may be encountered are reviewed subsequently. The organ-and-disease panels shown in Table 12–5 (p. 198) provide a source of focused testing in selected patients.

Glycemia: Glucose and Hemoglobin A_{1c}

Elevated plasma glucose measurement results (e.g., above a reference fasting interval concentration between 50 and 110 mg/dL) are associated with many syndromes and diseases. Some of these are shown in Table 12–6 and separated into primary (diabetes mellitus) and secondary causes (p. 199).

Hemoglobin A_{1c} ($<7\%$) or glycosylated hemoglobin is also used to monitor patients for long-term glucose control in the management of diabetes mellitus and to confirm hyperglycemia without apparent explanation. Validity of hemoglobin A_{1c} determinations is in part method dependent. However, they reflect blood glucose concentrations during the 120-day life span of the red blood cell. As methodology is refined further, hemoglobin A_{1c} may have future use as a determination for case finding and diagnosis as well as management for diabetes mellitus. Causes of hypoglycemia (<50 mg/dL of plasma, fasting, overnight specimen) are shown in Table 12–7 (p. 200).

Table 12–2 □ **GUIDE TO SUGGESTED SPECIMEN COLLECTION**

Chemistry (7-mL plain red top tube)
  Acetaminophen (μg/mL)
  Acetone
  Albumin (g/dL)
  Alanine aminotransferase
    (ALT; U/L)
  Alkaline phosphatase
    (U/L @ 37°C)
  Amylase (U/L)
  Aspartate aminotransferase
    (AST; U/L)
  Barbiturate screen
  Bilirubin (mg/gL)
  Blood urea nitrogen
    (BUN; mg/dL)
  Calcium (mEq/L)
  Calcium, ionized (mmol/L)
  Carbamazepine (μg/mL)
  CEA (ng/mL)
  Chloride, sweat (mmol/L)
  Cholesterol (mg/dL)
  Cortisol (μg/dL)
  Creatine kinase (CK; U/L)
  CKMB (ng/mL)
  Creatinine (mg/dL)
  Cyclosporine (ng/mL)
  Digoxin (ng/mL)
  Electrolytes (mmol/L)
    Chloride
    CO_2
    Potassium
    Sodium
  Ethosuximide
    (Zarontin; μg/mL)
  Ethanol (do not use
    alcohol swabs)
  Ferritin (ng/mL)
  Follicle-stimulating hormone
    (mIU/mL)
  Folic acid (ng/mL)
  Free thyroxine (free T_4)
  Gentamicin (μg/mL)
  Glucose (mg/dL)
  Growth hormone (ng/mL)
  hCG (mIU/L)
  Hemoglobin A_{1c} (%)
  Iron (μg/dL)
  Lactic acid (mmol/L)

  Lactate dehydrogenase
    (LD; U/L)
  Luteinizing hormone
    (LH; mU/mL)
  Lithium (mmol/L)
  Lipase (U/L)
  Magnesium (mEq/L)
  Osmolality, serum (mOsm/kg)
  Phenobarbital (μg/mL)
  Phenytoin (Dilantin; μg/mL)
  Phosphorus (mg/dL)
  Primidone (μg/mL)
  Procainamide (μg/mL)
  Prolactin (ng/dL)
  Prostate-specific antigen
    (ng/mL)
  Protein (g/dL)
  Salicylate (mg/dL)
  Theophylline (μg/mL)
  Thiocyanate (mg/dL)
  Tobramycin (μg/mL)
  Thyroid-stimulating hormone
    (μU/mL)
  Triglyceride (mg/dL)
  Triiodothyronine (T_3; ng/dL)
  Thyroxine (T_4; μg/mL)
  Uric acid (mg/dL)
  Valproic acid (μg/mL)
  Vancomycin (mg/dL)
  Vitamin B_{12} (pg/mL)
  Zinc (μg/mL)
Heparin (5-mL green top tube)
  Ammonia (on ice; μmol/L)
  Carboxyhemoglobin/O_2
    saturation
  Methemoglobin
  Hemoglobin, plasma (mg/dL)
NaF oxalate (5-mL gray
  top tube)
  Glucose
  Glucose tolerance
  Lactate (on ice)
  Lactose tolerance
EDTA (Versene; 7-mL
  lavender top tube)
  Carcinoembryonic antigen
    (CEA; ng/mL)
  Lead (μg/dL)

Table 12–2 □ GUIDE TO SUGGESTED SPECIMEN
COLLECTION *Continued*

Immunology	Heparin (7-mL green top tube)
Plain tube (7-mL red top tube)	Lymphocyte subsets
All antibody tests	Lymphoma/leukemia panel
EDTA (Versene; 7-mL	Nitroblue tetrazolium (NBT)
lavender top tube)	Phagocytosis (2 tubes)
Lymphocyte subsets	

From Henry JB: Clinical Diagnosis and Management by Laboratory Methods, 19th ed. Philadelphia, WB Saunders Co, 1996, p 14.

Two to three tests can be done per tube, unless otherwise specified.

CEA = Carcinoembryonic antigen; CKMB = creatine kinase MB isoenzyme; hCG = human chorionic gonadotropin; U = units.

Nitrogen Exchange Coins: BUN, Creatinine, and Uric Acid

The major coins of nitrogen exchange include blood urea nitrogen (BUN), creatinine, and uric acid. In renal failure, there is an initial elevation of BUN followed subsequently (from hours to days) by creatinine in proportion to muscle mass and lastly by a uric acid elevation. Urea is the more dialyzable moiety, and thus its blood concentration will reflect dialysis procedures, whereas plasma creatinine may not and is less helpful in infants, the elderly, and others with diminished muscle mass. Plasma uric acid is uniquely elevated in patients with eclampsia and of course in patients with gout.

Table 12–3 □ COLOR-CODED TUBE SELECTION
OF ANTICOAGULANTS COMMONLY USED

Stopper Color	Additive	Notes
Red	No additive	Collection of serum
Lavender	EDTA (Versene)	Collection of whole blood; binds calcium
Green	Heparin	Inhibits thrombin activation
Blue	Buffered citrate	Coagulation studies: binds calcium
Black	Buffered sodium citrate	Westergren ESR
Gray	Contains glycolytic inhibitor for glucose	Glucose determinations
Yellow	Citrate dextrose (ACD)	Preserves red cells

From Henry JB: Clinical Diagnosis and Management by Laboratory Methods, 19th ed. Philadelphia, WB Saunders Co, 1996, p 13.

Text continued on page 198

Table 12–4 □ SOME DRUGS WITH PHYSIOLOGIC EFFECTS ON OR CHEMICAL INTERFERENCE WITH COMMONLY ORDERED CONSTITUENTS IN BLOOD AND URINE

	Drugs Causing Physiologic Effect	Type of Effect*	Drugs with Chemical Interference	Type of Effect*
CONSTITUENT IN BLOOD				
Acid phosphatase (ACP)	Androgens (in women)	I	Fluorides	D
			Oxalates	D
Alkaline phosphatase (ALP)	Phenytoin	I	Albumin from placental sources	—
			Fluorides	D
			Oxalates	D
			Theophylline	D
			Isoniazid	—
Ammonia			Citrate	D
			Oxalate	D
			Fluorides	D
Amylase (AMS)	Cholinergics	—	Dextran	—
	Ethanol	—	Novobiocin	—
	Narcotics	—		
Bilirubin	Chlordiazepoxide	—	Ascorbic acid	—
	Gallbladder dyes	—	Caffeine	D
	Phenobarbital	D	Theophylline	D
			Heparin	D
Bromsulphalein (BSP)	Barbiturate	—	Phenazopyridine	—
	Clofibrate	—	Phenolphthalein	—
	Narcotics (opiates—meperidine and methadone)	—	Phenolsulfonphthalein	—
	Phenytoin	—		
	Probenecid	—		

Analyte	Substance	Effect
Calcium	Androgens	I
	Calciferol-activated calcium salts	I
	Citrate salts	D
	EDTA (interferes with dye-binding methods)	D
	Dihydrotachysterol	—
	Progestins-estrogens	—
	Thiazide diuretics	—
	Acetazolamide	D
	Corticosteroids	D
	Mithramycin	D
Chloride	Acetazolamides	—
	Chlorides	—
	Oxyphenbutazone	—
	Phenylbutazone	—
	Bromide	I
	ACTH, corticosteroids	D
	Ethacrynic acid	D
	Furosemide	D
	Mercurial diuretics	D
	Triamterene	D
Cholesterol	ACTH	—
	Bile salts	—
	Chlorpromazine	—
	Bromide	I
	Heparin	D
	Thyroxine	D
Cortisol	Chlordiazepoxide	—
	Dexamethasone	—
	Digoxin	—
	Methenamine	—
	Thorazine	—

Table continued on following page

Table 12–4 □ SOME DRUGS WITH PHYSIOLOGIC EFFECTS ON OR CHEMICAL INTERFERENCE WITH COMMONLY ORDERED CONSTITUENTS IN BLOOD AND URINE *Continued*

	Drugs Causing Physiologic Effect	Type of Effect*	Drugs with Chemical Interference	Type of Effect*
CONSTITUENT IN BLOOD *Continued*				
Creatine kinase (CK)	Carbenoxolone	—		
	Clofibrate	—		
	Codeine	—		
	Dexamethasone	—		
	Digoxin	—		
	Ethanol	—		
	Furosemide	—		
	Glutethimide	—		
	Halothane anesthesia	—		
	Heroin	—		
	Imipramine	—		
	Lithium carbonate	—		
	Meperidine hydrochloride	—		
	Morphine sulfate	—		
	Phenobarbital	—		
	Suxamethonium	—		
Creatinine	Amphotericin B	—	Ascorbic acid	—
	Kanamycin	—	Barbiturates	—
			Cephalosporins	—
			Glucose	—
			Levodopa	—

Analyte	Drug	Effect
Creatinine *Continued*	Methyldopa	I
	BSP and phenolsulfonphthalein	I
Glucose	ACTH, corticosteroids	I
	Epinephrine	I
	Ethacrynic acid	—
	Furosemide	—
	Phenytoin	—
	Propranolol	D
	Acetaminophen	—
	Aminosalicylic acid (*para*-aminosalicylic acid)	—
	Ascorbic acid	—
	Dextran	I or D
	Isoproterenol	—
	Levodopa	—
	Mercaptopurine	—
	Methimazole	—
	Methyldopa	—
	Nalidixic acid	—
	Oxazepam	—
	Propylthiouracil	—
	Hydralazine	—
Lactate dehydrogenase	Thiazides	I
	Clofibrate	D
	Oxalate	D
Lipase	Cholinergics	—
	Ethanol	—
	Narcotics	—
	Calciferol-activated methicillin	—
	Tetracyclines	—
	Theophylline	D
Phosphate	Aluminum hydroxide	D
	Glucose infusion	D
	Insulin	D
	Mithramycin	D
	Bilirubin	—

Table continued on following page

Table 12–4 □ SOME DRUGS WITH PHYSIOLOGIC EFFECTS ON OR CHEMICAL INTERFERENCE WITH COMMONLY ORDERED CONSTITUENTS IN BLOOD AND URINE *Continued*

	Drugs Causing Physiologic Effect	Type of Effect*	Drugs with Chemical Interference	Type of Effect*
CONSTITUENT IN BLOOD *Continued*				
Potassium	Heparin	I	Calcium	I
	Potassium	I	Penicillin G	I
	Spironolactone	I		
	ACTH, corticosteroids	D		
	Amphotericin	D		
	Glucose infusion	D		
	Insulin	D		
	Oral diuretics	D		
	Salicylates	D		
	Tetracycline	D		
Protein (total protein)	ACTH, corticosteroids	I	BSP dye	I
	Anabolic/androgenic steroids	I	Bilirubin	I
			Dextran	I
			Phenazopyridine	I
			Acetylsalicylic acid	D
Sodium	Androgens	I		
	Rauwolfia alkaloids	I		
	Corticosteroids	I		
	Mannitol	I		
	Methyldopa	I		
	Oxyphenbutazone	I		

Sodium *Continued*

Substance	
Phenylbutazone	—
Ammonium chloride	D
Heparin	D
Oral diuretics	D
Mercurial diuretics	D
Spironolactone	D

Transferases
AST (GOT) and ALT (GPT)

Substance	
Ampicillin	—
Cephalothin	—
Clofibrate	—
Colchicine	—
Gentamicin	—
Methyltestosterone	—
Nafcillin	—
Opiates	—
Oxacillin	—

For spectrophotometric assay of AST:

Substance	
Ascorbic acid	—
Erythromycin	—
Isoniazid	—
Levodopa	—
para-Aminosalicylic acid (PAS)	—

Urate

Substance	
Adrenocortical steroids	—
Busulfan	—
Ethacrynic acid	—
Nitrogen mustard	—
Purine analogue antimetabolites	—
Pyrazinamide	—
Quinethazone	—
Thiazides	—
Vincristine sulfate	—
Acetylsalicylic acid	D
Allopurinol	D
Chlorpromazine	D
Ascorbic acid	—
Glucose	—
Methyldopa	—
Theophylline	—

Table continued on following page

Table 12–4 □ SOME DRUGS WITH PHYSIOLOGIC EFFECTS ON OR CHEMICAL INTERFERENCE WITH COMMONLY ORDERED CONSTITUENTS IN BLOOD AND URINE *Continued*

Drugs Causing Physiologic Effect	Type of Effect*	Drugs with Chemical Interference	Type of Effect*
CONSTITUENT IN BLOOD *Continued*			
Urate Continued			
Chlorprothixene	D		
Oxyphenbutazone	D		
Phenylbutazone	D		
Probenecid	D		
		Chloral hydrate	—
		Chlorobutanol	—
		Guanethidine	—
Urea			
Alkaline antacids	—		
Antimony salts	—		
Arsenicals	—		
Cephaloridine	—		
Furosemide	—		
Gentamicin	—		
Kanamycin	—		
Methyldopa	—		
Neomycin	—		
CONSTITUENT IN URINE			
Catecholamines			
Nitroglycerin	—	B vitamin (high dose)	—
Phenothiazines	—	Erythromycin	—
MAO inhibitors	D	Hydralazine	—
		Levodopa	—
		Methenamine hippurate	—
		Methenamine mandelate	—

Catecholamines *Continued*		
	Methyldopa	I
	Nicotinic acid	—
	Quinine-quinidine	—
	Salicylate	—
	Tetracyclines	—
	Bromide	—
	Ascorbic acid	—
	Levodopa	—
	Methyldopa	—
	Nitrofuran derivatives	—
Chloride		
Creatinine		
Glucose		
1. Enzymatic method (Clinistix, Tes Tape)	Ascorbic acid	D
	Levodopa	D
2. Benedict's solution of Clinitest	Ascorbic acid	—
	Cephalosporins	—
	Chloral hydrate	—
	Nitrofuran derivatives	—
	Mephenesin	—
	Methocarbamol	—
	Phenothiazines	D
Hydroxyindoleacetic acid (5-HIAA)	Reserpine	I
17-Hydroxycorticosteroids (17-OH)		
17-Ketogenic steroids (17-KGS)		
17-Ketosteroids (17-KS)		
17-KS	Anabolic steroids	—
17-KS, 17-OH	Phenytoin	D
17-KS, 17-OH	Estrogens	D

Table continued on following page

Table 12–4 □ SOME DRUGS WITH PHYSIOLOGIC EFFECTS ON OR CHEMICAL INTERFERENCE WITH COMMONLY ORDERED CONSTITUENTS IN BLOOD AND URINE *Continued*

	Drugs Causing Physiologic Effect	Type of Effect*	Drugs with Chemical Interference	Type of Effect*
CONSTITUENT IN URINE *Continued*				
17-KS	Ethacrynic acid	D		
17-KS, 17-KGS	Penicillin	D		
17-KS	Probenecid	D		
17-OH	Thiazide diuretics	D		
17-OH, 17-KS, 17-KGS	Meprobamate	—		
17-OH, 17-KS, 17-KGS	Phenothiazines	—		
17-OH, 17-KS, 17-KGS	Spironolactone	—		
17-OH, 17-KS, 17-KGS	Penicillin G	—		
17-OH	Ascorbic acid	—		
17-OH	Chloral hydrate	—		
17-OH	Chlordiazepoxide	—		
17-OH	Hydroxyzine	—		
17-OH	Inorganic iodides	—		
17-OH	Methenamine	—		
17-KS			Phenothiazines	—
17-OH			Quinidine, quinine	—

Test	Drug	Effect*
17-OH	Reserpine	D
17-KS	Ethinamate	D
17-OH, 17-KS, 17-KGS	Nalidixic acid	
Phenolsulfonphthalein	Penicillin	D
	Probenecid	D
	Salicylates	D
	Sulfonamides	D
	Thiazide diuretics	D
	Progestins-estrogens	I
Porphyrins	Acriflavine	I
	Ethoxazene	I
	Phenazopyridine	I
	Procaine	I
	Sulfonamides	I
	Mandelamine	I
	Anileridine	I
	Caffeine	I
	Mandelamine	I
	Methocarbamol	I
	Salicylates	I
Pregnanediol		
Vanillylmandelic acid	Epinephrine	I
	Lithium carbonate	I
	Nitroglycerin	I
	Chlorpromazine	D
	Guanethidine	D
	MAO inhibitors	D
	Reserpine	D

Modified from Martin TJ: The Pharmacologic Interactions with Laboratory Test Values. Washington, DC, Bureau of Standards, Circular 547, US Department of Commerce, 1954; and Young DS, Pestaner LC, Gibberman V: Clin Chem 1975; 21:1D.
*I indicates an increase and D a decrease.

Table 12–5 □ ORGAN/DISEASE PANELS COMPOSITION AND CURRENT PROCEDURAL TERMINOLOGY CODES (YEAR 2000)

1. Basic metabolic panel—80048
   Glucose—82947
   Calcium—82310
   Creatinine—82565
   Urea nitrogen (BUN)—84520
   Sodium—84295
   Potassium—84132
   Carbon dioxide—82374
   Chloride—82435

2. Comprehensive metabolic panel
   —80053
   AST, SGOT—84450
   ALT, SGPT—84460
   Bilirubin, total—82247
   Phosphatase, alkaline—84075
   Protein, total—84155
   Albumin—82040
   Glucose—82947
   BUN—84520
   Creatinine—82565
   Sodium—84295
   Potassium—84132
   Chloride—82435
   Carbon dioxide—82374
   Calcium—82310

3. Hepatic function panel—80076
   Transferase, aspartate amino
      (AST) (SGOT)—84450
   Transferase, alanine amino
      (ALT) (SGPT)—84460
   Phosphatase, alkaline—84075
   Bilirubin, total—82247
   Bilirubin, direct—82248
   Protein, total—84155
   Albumin—82040

4. Acute hepatitis panel—80074
   Hepatitis B surface antigen
      (HBsAg)—87340
   Hepatitis B core antibody
      (HBcAb), IgM antibody
      —86705
   Hepatitis C antibody—86803
   Hepatitis A antibody (HAAb), IgM
      antibody—86709

5. Renal function panel—80069
   Creatinine—82565
   Urea nitrogen (BUN)—84520
   Calcium—82310
   Phosphorus, inorganic
      (phosphate)—84100
   Sodium—84295
   Potassium—84132
   Carbon dioxide—82374
   Chloride—82435
   Albumin—82040
   Glucose—82947

6. Electrolyte panel—80051
   Carbon dioxide—82374
   Chloride—82435
   Potassium—84132
   Sodium—84295

CPT Codes © American Medical Association

The most common cause of a low plasma BUN in hospitalized patients is overhydration, and mild elevations are observed with dehydration and gastrointestinal hemorrhage. Compared with urea, plasma creatinine concentrations are considered a better indicator of glomerular function. The ratio of BUN to serum creatinine is generally between 10:1 and 20:1. With renal parenchymal damage or reduction (>50%), BUN and creatinine rise in concert and

Table 12–6 □ CLASSIFICATION OF HYPERGLYCEMIA

Primary
    Insulin-dependent diabetes mellitus
    Non-insulin-dependent diabetes mellitus
Secondary
    Hyperglycemia resulting from disease of the pancreas
        Inflammation
            Acute pancreatitis (rare)
            Chronic pancreatitis
            Pancreatitis due to mumps
            ? Cell damage due to coxsackievirus B4 infection
            ? Autoimmune disease
        Pancreatectomy
        Pancreatic infiltration
            Hemochromatosis
            Tumors
        Trauma to pancreas (rare)
    Hyperglycemia related to other major endocrine diseases
        Acromegaly
        Cushing's syndrome
        Thyrotoxicosis
        Pheochromocytoma
        Hyperaldosteronism
        Glucagonoma
        Somatostatinoma
    Hyperglycemia caused by drugs
        Steroids
        Thiazide diuretics, propranolol, phenytoin, and diazoxide
        Oral contraceptives
        Alloxan and streptozotocin
    Hyperglycemia related to other major disease states
        Chronic renal failure
        Chronic liver disease
        Infection
    Miscellaneous hyperglycemia
        Pregnancy
        Related to insulin receptor antibodies (acanthosis nigricans)
        Abnormal insulin

From Henry JB: Clinical Diagnosis and Management by Laboratory Methods, 19th ed. Philadelphia, WB Saunders Co, 1996, p 198.

maintain a similar ratio. One assay (creatinine) thus may confirm the implications of the other (BUN), with the ratio (BUN/creatinine) being suggestive of a cause. Compromised renal blood flow results in a low urine flow rate and enhanced urea reabsorption without decreasing creatinine secretion proportionately. Low urine flow may be attributable to dehydration, cardiac pump failure with congestive heart failure, hepatorenal syndrome, or urinary tract obstruction, e.g., prostatic nodular hyperplasia. A serum

Table 12–7 □ CLASSIFICATION OF SOME OF THE MORE COMMON CAUSES OF HYPOGLYCEMIA

No anatomic lesion present
  Fasting plasma glucose normal
    Reactive hypoglycemia
      Functional hypoglycemia
      Alimentary hypoglycemia
      Diabetic and impaired glucose tolerance
  Fasting plasma glucose low
    Ethanol-induced hypoglycemia
    Drug-induced hypoglycemia
      Sulfonylurea
      Phenformin*
      Insulin
      Ethanol
      Salicylates
      Combinations of the above
    Factitious—fasting glucose normal or low
Anatomic lesion present
  Insulinoma
  Extrapancreatic neoplasms
  Adrenocortical insufficiency
  Hypopituitarism
  Massive liver disease

From Henry JB: Clinical Diagnosis and Management by Laboratory Methods, 19th ed. Philadelphia, WB Saunders Co, 1996, p 199.
*No longer available in the United States.

creatinine value divided into 1 is a guide to approximate glomerular flow rate (GFR), or creatinine clearance (e.g., $1 \div 2.0$ mg/dL creatinine = 50%). Acute renal failure causes are shown in Table 13–1 (p. 235), and helpful hints to evaluate patients with oliguria are shown in Table 12–8.

Calcium and Phosphate

As the most abundant cation in the body, calcium is stored in bone as hydroxyapatite and hydroxyphosphate with an equilibrium between insoluble calcium phosphate and soluble calcium phosphate.

$$K_{sp} = [Ca] \times [P] \div CaP \text{ insoluble}$$

When the K_{sp}, or solubility product constant, is exceeded, calcium can precipitate, i.e., undergo calcinosis. There is an inverse relationship between [Ca] and [P] plasma values. Hypercalcemic states are almost always accompanied by hypophosphatemia and vice versa. Furthermore, soluble calcium (in the numerator) in blood is in two forms, one bound to albumin and globulin

Table 12–8 □ HELPFUL LABORATORY EVALUATIONS TO ASSESS OLIGURIA

Diagnostic Test	Prerenal	Renal	Postrenal
Urine volume	<500 mL/day	<500 mL/day	Variable
BUN/creatinine ratio in serum	>20:1	10:1	Variable
Urine/plasma urea concentration	>10:1	<10:1	About 15:1
Urine/plasma creatinine concentration	>20:1	<20:1	<20:1
Urine specific gravity	>1.020	About 1.010	About 1.010
Urine osmolality	>600 mOsm/kg	About 300 mOsm/kg	About 300 mOsm/kg
Urine/plasma osmolality	>2:1	<12:1	Variable
Urine sodium concentration	<20 mEq/L	>30 mEq/L	>30 mEq/L
Fractional excretion Na	>1.0	>1.0	>1.0
Renal failure index	>1.0	>1.0	>1.0

$$\text{Fractional excretion Na} = \frac{[\text{urine Na}] \times [\text{plasma creatinine}]}{[\text{plasma Na}] \times [\text{urine creatinine}]} \times 100$$

$$\text{Renal failure index} = \frac{[\text{urine Na}] \times [\text{plasma creatinine}]}{[\text{urine creatinine}]} \times 100$$

From Henry JB: Clinical Diagnosis and Management by Laboratory Methods, 19th ed. Philadelphia, WB Saunders Co, 1996, p 149.

(chelated) and the other ionized (nonchelated). Hence, the plasma-ionized calcium (1.13 to 1.32 mEq/L) as opposed to the total calcium (4.2 to 5.1 mEq/L) measurement is preferable to reflect biologically active calcium. Ionized-calcium assays do not reflect the vagaries of hyperproteinemia and hypoproteinemia and thus are more clinically relevant in such patients with multiple myeloma or polyclonal gammopathy.

In renal disease, tubular failure causes phosphate excretion to be inhibited (the tubules are nonresponsive to parathyroid hormone), and this inhibition gives rise to decreasing calcium and increasing phosphate levels. Hypocalcemia and hyperphosphatemia in the presence of azotemia (elevated BUN and creatinine) indicate renal disease and point to tubular failure.

Other causes of hypocalcemia to keep in mind, besides alkalemia and renal failure, are hypoparathyroidism and rarely medullary thyroid carcinoma and other tumors with elaboration of calcitonin. Likewise, hypercalcemia is observed in acidemia, metastatic carcinoma, multiple myeloma, sarcoidosis, hyperparathyroidism, and iatrogenic conditions.

Magnesium

The magnesium cation is an essential mineral and the fourth most-abundant cation in humans. Magnesium in the salt or free ion form (as opposed to the nonionic form) is most important. Magnesium is also a cofactor in numerous intracellular enzymatic reactions, e.g., phosphate transfer from ADP and ATP in muscle contractility and neuronal transmission. The majority of magnesium in the human body is located in the bones (~50%) in the form of phosphates and carbonates and in soft tissues, with the remainder being found principally in the liver and muscles; red blood cells also contain magnesium. Magnesium inhibits nerve impulses and relaxes muscle contractions, thereby functioning antagonistically to calcium. On the other hand, like calcium, magnesium can bind phosphates and can substitute for calcium as a bone or tooth mineral. Although its physiologic role is primarily intracellular, assays for total and ionized magnesium in plasma-serum and whole blood are most helpful in elucidating plasma electrolyte abnormalities, especially with a low potassium level that appears refractory to replacement therapy. Magnesium deficiency is observed postoperatively and in association with severe and sustained stress. It may also enhance the immune response, clarify electrocardiographic abnormalities, and be a contributing factor in arrhythmias.

About one third of total serum magnesium (1.3 to 2.1 mEq/L, or 0.7 to 1.1 mmol/L) is bound to protein (mostly albumin), and the other two thirds is ultrafiltrable, predominantly the free ion with a small percentage as a complex of ions.

Magnesium depletion is often overlooked in hospitalized patients. Manifestations include weakness, muscle fasciculations, agitation, depression, seizures, hypocalcemia, hypokalemia, and cardiac arrhythmias. It may be present in alcoholism, early chronic renal failure, hemodialysis, digitalis intoxication, pregnancy at term (eclampsia with toxemia), diuretic therapy, porphyria, and Paget's disease.

Hypermagnesemia is also not uncommon. Signs of magnesium toxicity include anesthesia, flaccidity, paralysis of the voluntary muscles, and hypotension. It may be caused by advanced renal failure, Addison's disease, severe dehydration, acute diabetic ketoacidosis, and excessive administration of magnesium sulfate.

Electrolytes and Acid-Base Balance

Results of electrolytes (Na^+, K^+, Cl^-, and HCO_3^- as total CO_2) are often a challenge, especially in hyponatremia and hypernatremia (Tables 12–9 and 12–10). Blood pH most often with blood gas measurements defines acidemia (<7.40) and alkalemia (>7.40), or acid-base status (Table 12–11). The bicarbonate or the P_{CO_2} can then be used to delineate metabolic or respiratory origin (Table 12–12); the pH of blood can also affect the levels of electrolytes in plasma or serum. The bicarbonate/carbonic acid equilibrium is as follows:

$$H_2O + CO_2 \rightleftharpoons H_2CO_3 \rightleftharpoons H^+ + HCO_3^-$$

It is expressed in the following equations, which assist in the analysis of acid-base disturbances:

$$pH = pK_a + \log \frac{[HCO_3^-]}{H_2CO_3}$$

$$pH = pK_a' + \log \frac{(Total\ CO_2) - 0.03\ P_{CO_2}}{0.03\ P_{CO_2}}$$

$$[H^+]\ nmol/L = \frac{24\ P_{CO_2}\ (mm\ Hg)}{[HCO_3^-]\ mmol/L}$$

In acidemia, red blood cells and proteins, after bicarbonate and phosphates, buffer excess H^+ ions by exchanging for intracellular K^+ with a net hyperkalemia often seen with a mild hypercalcemia. Hypokalemia occurs in alkalemia often with depressed ionized-calcium values.

The anion gap (AG) is depicted in Fig. 12–1, which shows the difference between anions and cations routinely measured in plasma, i.e., Na^+, K^+, Cl^-, and HCO_3^- (as total CO_2). Unmeasured cations usually are calcium and magnesium (averaging 7 mmol/L), whereas unmeasured anions include phosphate, sulfate,

Table 12–9 □ COMMON CAUSES OF HYPONATREMIA AND ELECTROLYTE PATTERNS IN SERUM AND URINE WITH NORMAL RENAL FUNCTION*

Cause	Serum Na	Urine Na	Urine Osm	Serum K	24-Hour UNa
1. Overhydration	Low	Low	Low	Normal or low	Low
2. Diuretics	Low	Low	Low	Low	High
3. SIADH	Low	High	High	Normal or low	High
4. Adrenal failure	Low	Mildly elevated	Normal	High	High
5. Bartter's syndrome	Low	Low	Low	Low	High

From Henry JB: Clinical Diagnosis and Management by Laboratory Methods, 19th ed. Philadelphia, WB Saunders Co, 1996, p 82.
*All Na and K values are concentrations except for 24-hour UNa, which is the total number of milliequivalents of Na excreted in 24 hours in the urine.
SIADH, secretion of inappropriate levels of antidiuretic hormone.

Table 12–10 □ COMMON CAUSES OF HYPERNATREMIA AND ELECTROLYTE PATTERNS IN SERUM AND URINE WITH NORMAL RENAL FUNCTION*

Cause	Serum Na	Urine Na	Urine Osm	Serum K	24-Hour UNa
1. Dehydration	High	High	High	Normal	Low
2. Diabetes insipidus	High	Low	Low	Normal	Low
3. Cushing's disease or syndrome	High	Low	Normal	Low	Low

From Henry JB: Clinical Diagnosis and Management by Laboratory Methods, 19th ed. Philadelphia, WB Saunders Co, 1996, p 83.
*In this table, low is equivalent to depressed, and high is equivalent to elevated. All Na and K values are concentrations except for 24-hour UNa, which is the total number of milliequivalents of Na excreted in 24 hours in the urine.

Table 12–11 □ THE BICARBONATE BUFFER SYSTEM

$H^+ + HCO_3^- = H_2CO_3 = CO_2 + H_2O$
Why is normal $[H^+]$ 40 nmol/L?

Normal acid-base values

Blood $Pa_{CO_2} = 38 - 42$ mm Hg
Plasma $HCO_3^- = 24 - 28$ mmol/L

Henderson equation

$$[H^+] \text{ (nmol/L)} = \frac{24 \ P_{CO_2} \text{ (mm Hg)}}{HCO_3^- \text{ (mmol/L)}}$$

$$[H^+] = \frac{24 \times 40}{24} = 40 \text{ nmol/L}$$

From Henry JB: Clinical Diagnosis and Management by Laboratory Methods, 19th ed. Philadelphia, WB Saunders Co, 1996, p 150.

protein, and organic acids (all averaging less than 24 mmol/L). The sum of sodium and potassium minus chloride and total CO_2 yields an anion gap of ~140 − 124 = 16 mEq/L as other counteranions that neutralize sodium but are not measured regularly.

In metabolic acidemia in which acid is retained (HCl), the bicarbonate value decreases, but there is a 1:1 increase in chloride, and so the anion gap does not change. If metabolic acidemia is caused by other fixed acids (acetoacetic acid in diabetic acidosis or lactic acid in sepsis, uremia, or hypoperfusion), bicarbonate is reduced without a corresponding increment in chloride. Hence there is an increase in the anion gap (25 to 30 mEq/L). A widened anion gap is indicative of metabolic acidemia caused by a non-chloride containing acid. Suspect an organic acidemia when the anion gap exceeds 30 mEq/L. A decreased anion gap (<10 or typically 1 to 3) may be observed in hyperproteinemia (myeloma and polyclonal gammopathy), hypermagnesemia, and lithium intoxication.

Arterial Blood Gas Pattern

Tissue perfusion and pulmonary diffusion (alveolar capillary block) are reflected in P_{O_2} (90 to 100 mm Hg), shown in Fig. 12–2 as the oxygen-hemoglobin dissociation curve. Hypoxemia may be associated with pulmonary diffusion lesions or defects or decreased blood perfusion (pulmonary infarction or lung collapse with atelectasis) in association with several different acute and chronic pulmonary and cardiac (pump) failure diseases. The plasma P_{CO_2} is usually normal, or it may be depressed with hyperventilation as a result of hypoxemia and associated acidemia (lactic acid from decreased tissue perfusion).

Table 12-12 □ PATTERNS OF pH, P_{CO_2}, AND BICARBONATE IN DIFFERENT CONDITIONS

Condition	pH	Bicarbonate	P_{CO_2}	Typical Causes
1. Metabolic acidosis	<7.40	Low	Low	Diabetic ketoacidosis; lactic acidosis
2. Metabolic alkalosis	>7.40	High	High	Vomiting
3. Respiratory acidosis	<7.40	High	High	COPD; paralysis of respiratory muscles
4. Respiratory alkalosis	>7.40	Low	Low	Anxiety; acute pain

From Henry JB: Clinical Diagnosis and Management by Laboratory Methods, 19th ed. Philadelphia, WB Saunders Co, 1996, p 85. COPD, chronic obstructive pulmonary disease.

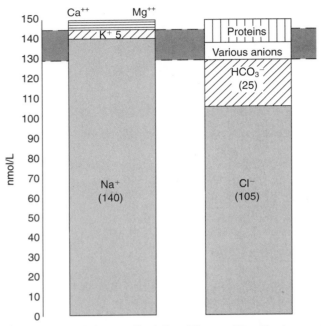

Figure 12–1 □ Anion gap. Depiction of the quantities of anions and cations in the circulating blood. The positive charges equal the negative charges to maintain electrical neutrality. However, only Na^+, K^+, Cl^-, and HCO_3^- are routinely measured. The sum of the measured positive charges (Na^+, K^+) *(top interrupted line)* normally exceeds the sum of the measured negative charges (Cl^- + HCO_3^-) *(bottom interrupted line)*. This difference, which is known as the anion gap, is depicted by *shading* outside the histogram. (From Henry JB: Clinical Diagnosis and Management by Laboratory Methods, 19th ed. Philadelphia, WB Saunders Co, 1996, p 151.)

CO_2 retention states such as severe COPD (chronic obstructive pulmonary disease or emphysema) allow CO_2 to build up in alveoli, reducing O_2 in the alveolar air space. When the PCO_2 exceeds 50 mm Hg, the effect on alveolar PO_2 is shown in Fig. 12–3. O_2, unlike CO_2, is not soluble in water including membranes, and so there is a difference of about 10 to 15 mm Hg between alveolar (A) O_2 and arterial (a) O_2, also called the "A-a gradient," expressed as follows:

$$P_AO_2 - P_aO_2 = 10 \text{ mm Hg}$$

A pattern of low arterial blood pH, low PO_2, low oxygen saturation, high PCO_2, and low bicarbonate is unlike the four basic pat-

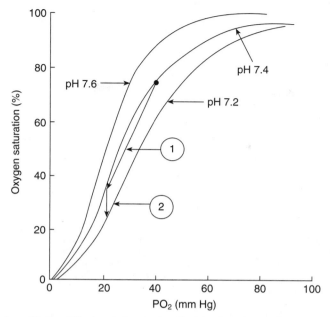

Figure 12–2 □ Effects of decreasing P_{O_2} in the allosteric zone of the oxygen-hemoglobin dissociation curve. On the pH 7.4 curve, if the P_{O_2} drops from 80 to 60, there is little effect on the oxygen saturation. However, a drop from 40 to 20 mm Hg results in a large drop in oxygen saturation from about 80% to 30% *(arrow 1)*. With this low oxygen saturation, there is a significant tissue lactic acidosis from anaerobic metabolism. The increased acidosis results in a drop in blood pH to 7.2, shifting the oxygen-hemoglobin dissociation to the right (pH 7.2 curve). Now, for a P_{O_2} of 30, the oxygen saturation drops even further *(arrow 2)* to about 20%, setting a vicious cycle in motion. (From Henry JB: Clinical Diagnosis and Management by Laboratory Methods, 19th ed. Philadelphia, WB Saunders Co, 1996, p 86.)

terns shown in Table 12–12. On top of respiratory acidemia (high P_{CO_2}), there is a superimposed tissue metabolic lactic acidemia causing a low bicarbonate level, and associated low P_{O_2} should prompt ventilatory assistance. Administration of oxygen in such patients without ventilation can cause cessation of respiration and death.

Hepatic Function

Assessment of hepatocellular injury or necrosis and interference in bile canalicular flow is reflected in several proteins including

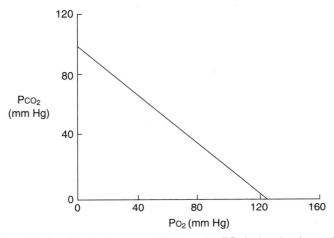

Figure 12–3 □ Effect of increased P_{CO_2} on the P_{O_2} in the alveolus and in arterial blood. This figure demonstrates that, as the P_{CO_2} increases, there is a greater than one-to-one decrease of P_{O_2}. (From Henry JB: Clinical Diagnosis and Management by Laboratory Methods, 19th ed. Philadelphia, WB Saunders Co, 1996, p 86.)

enzymes in the presence of acute or chronic hepatocyte injury or necrosis with subsequent fibrosis and scarring (cirrhosis). Interference with bile flow is manifest in bilirubin (total/direct) and alkaline phosphatase determinations. Gamma-glutamyl transferase (GGT) and 5′-nucleotidase (5′-N) are more specific and sensitive assays than alkaline phosphatase in measuring the interference in bile flow. Keep in mind, however, sensitivity of GGT to alcohol ingestion.

Six conditions and patterns are shown in Table 12–13 for a quick review.

Plasma protein changes (albumin depression secondary to decreased synthesis and with sustained stress) with polyclonal gammopathy including beta-gamma (β-γ) bridging are hallmarks of chronic liver disease. ALT > AST reflects hepatocyte injury or necrosis of acute liver disease. Albumin may also be considered a "reverse" acute-phase reactant.

Electrolyte, renal function, and coagulation abnormalities may also be observed. DIC (disseminated intravascular coagulation) may accompany liver failure as well as decreased coagulation factor production and thrombocytopenia (sequestration of platelets), especially in the presence of hepatosplenomegaly. An FSP (fibrin split products) or D-dimer assay when its results are elevated may clinch the diagnosis of DIC.

Table 12–13 □ SIX FUNDAMENTAL PATTERNS OF LIVER FUNCTION TESTS

Condition	AST	ALT	LD	ALP	TP	Alb	Bilirubin	Ammonia
1. Hepatitis	H	H	H	H	N	N	H	N
2. Cirrhosis	N	N	N	N-sl H	L	L	H	H
3. Biliary obstruction	N	N	N	H	N	N	H	
4. Space-occupying lesion	N or H	N or H	H	H	N	N	N-H	
5. Passive congestion	sl H	sl H	sl H	N-sl H	N	N	N-sl H	
6. Fulminant failure	very H	H	H	H	L	L	H	

From Henry JB: Clinical Diagnosis and Management by Laboratory Methods, 19th ed. Philadelphia, WB Saunders Co, 1996, p 87.
H. N. L. high, normal, low; AST, aspartate aminotransferase; ALT, alanine aminotransferase; LD, lactate dehydrogenase; ALP, alkaline phosphatase; TP, total protein, Alb, albumin; sl, Slightly.

trophoresis patterns can be diagnostic in
ιn help support the diagnosis in others.
ein components in serum is presented in
istinctive patterns are commonly seen
-5 and 12–6.

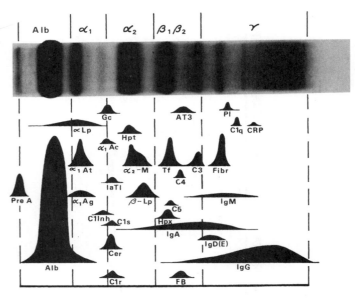

Figure 12–4 □ Plasma protein electrophoresis pattern in agarose gel is composed of five fractions, each composed of many individual species. Some of the major proteins are shown here in an artist's rendition for clarity.

α₁Ac = Alpha-1-antichymotrypsin
α₁Ag = Alpha-1-acid glycoprotein
α₁At = Alpha-1-antitrypsin
α₂-M = Alpha-2-macroglobulin
α-LP = Alpha lipoprotein
Alb = Albumin
AT3 = Antithrombin III
β-Lp = Beta-lipoprotein
Complement components:
  C1q, C1r, C1s, C3, C4,
  C5 = As designated
  C1Inh = C1 esterase inhibitor
Cer = Ceruloplasmin

CRP = C-reactive protein
Gc = Gc-globulin (vitamin D–
  binding protein)
FB = Factor B
Fibr = Fibrinogen
Hpt = Haptoglobin
Hpx = Hemopexin
Immunoglobulins: IgA, IgD, IgE,
  IgG, IgM = As designated
Pl = Plasminogen
Pre A = Prealbumin
Tf = Transferrin

(Modified from Laurell CB: Electrophoresis, specific protein assays, or both in measurement of plasma proteins? Con Chem 1973; 19:99.)

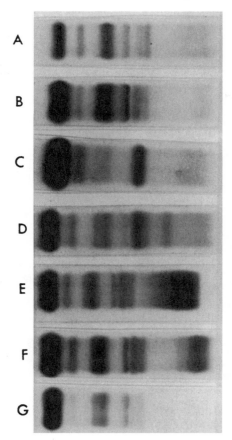

Figure 12–5 □ Abnormal protein patterns by agarose gel electrophoresis. Anode is to the left; fractions are as labeled in accord with those vertically in Figure 12–4; all samples are serum except for *C. A,* Inanition in an elderly patient with low total protein and greatly depressed albumin. *B,* Nephrotic syndrome with elevated alpha-2-macroglobulin and beta-lipoprotein. *C,* Urine from protein-losing nephropathy. *D,* Iron deficiency with elevated transferrin. *E,* Broadly elevated gamma globulin and low albumin because of liver disease. *F,* Oligoclonal gamma fraction in patient with renal disease. *G,* Hypogammaglobulinemia. (From Henry JB: Clinical Diagnosis and Management by Laboratory Methods, 19th ed. Philadelphia, WB Saunders Co, 1996, p 250.)

Detection of monoclonal bands in serum protein electrophoresis (SPEP) should prompt further immunofixation studies and quantitative immunoglobulin levels to establish the presence of a paraprotein. It is the responsibility of the resident in many instances to

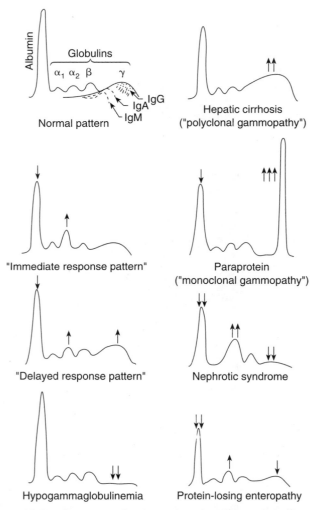

Figure 12–6 □ Serum protein electrophoresis: clinicopathologic correlations. (From Henry JB: Clinical Diagnosis and Management by Laboratory Methods, 19th ed. Philadelphia, WB Saunders Co, 1996, p 250; courtesy Dr. A.F. Krieg.)

follow up abnormal SPEPs. The clinician should be notified of the abnormal finding, and if it is a new development, orders for immunofixation studies and quantitative immunoglobulin levels should be obtained (this may be set up as reflexive testing, if allowed). Simultaneous urine protein determinations, urine protein electrophoresis, and immunofixation studies (if more than 15 mg/dL protein) may be appropriate in most instances. An unusual pitfall in the interpretation of urine protein electrophoresis arises in recipients of pancreatic transplants. The pancreatic duct is diverted into the bladder, and these patients usually have several prominent monoclonal bands, which represent pancreatic exocrine enzymes.

Ischemic Heart Disease

Salient features of laboratory determinations are reviewed in diagnosis and management of myocardial infarction. Total creatine kinase (CK) and in particular CK-MB mass elevation as a continuing rise or fall, with an increase in the ratio of CK-MB to total CK in serial assays, is pathognomonic of injured or necrotic myocardium, especially with CK-MB beginning to rise in 2 to 6 hours after the initial event and peaking within 12 hours (whereas total CK may not peak until 24 hours). Cardiac troponin I (cTnI), because of its greater specificity (expressed only in the heart), sensitivity, and duration of elevated value, is preferable and in combination with CK-MB in serial assays optimal for assessment of cardiac ischemic injury or necrosis. However, cTnI has displayed false elevations attributed to incomplete clotting of specimens (because of fibrin or hemolysis), heterophile antibodies, and chronic renal failure. A multispecific blocking reagent in two-site cTnI immunoassay may eliminate the interference caused by heterophile antibodies. Suspected false-positive sera cTnI assays should be confirmed with a plasma cTnI assay. Myoglobin elevation within 2 to 4 hours after AMI (acute myocardial infarction) but a return to normal by 12 to 24 hours after injury is the earliest-appearing marker with a high negative predictive value, whereas cTnI rises as early as 3 to 6 hours and is sustained for several (7 to 10) days (Fig. 12–7).

Hence, when calls arise from the Emergency Department and results do not fit the clinical picture, multiple markers should be measured serially (4- to 8-hour intervals) to clarify a false-positive result versus the onset of cardiac infarction. Clinical decisions to admit to the hospital or discharge a patient have to be made there in a timely manner.

Ischemic heart disease and coronary artery disease (CAD) association with acute inflammation may be substantiated with an increase in the patient's white blood cell count, platelet count, and elevated acute-phase reactants, e.g., alpha- and beta-globulins of serum proteins, fibrinogen, erythrocyte sedimentation rate (ESR), and C-reactive protein (CRP).

Coronary Artery Disease (CAD) Risk Factors

Lipid and lipoprotein measurements for assessment of risk factors in patients with suspected coronary artery heart disease

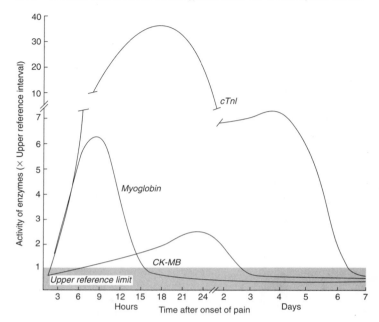

Figure 12–7 □ Typical serial measurements of CK-MB, myoglobin, and troponin-I (cTnI) pattern after the onset of acute myocardial infarction.

(CHD) are valuable to screen to detect persons at risk or case find to identify them, as in the following parameters:

- Total serum cholesterol, with precision and accuracy limits of ≳3%
- LDL ≳160 mg/dL
- LDL cholesterol ≳160 mg/dL
- HDL cholesterol <35 mg/dL and >60 mg/dL (risk protective)
- Triglycerides >200 mg/dL

Cholesterol as total and high-density-lipoprotein (HDL) cholesterol can be used to screen, detect, case find, or confirm patients at risk, and HDL cholesterol of <0.9 mmol/dL, or 35 mg/dL, is the low cutoff for identification of high-risk individuals. Hypertriglyceridemia (2.25 to 4.50 mmol/L, or 200 to 400 mg/dL) though borderline is associated with decreased HDL cholesterol levels observed in patients with CAD and diabetic patients.

Serum Lp(a), or lipoprotein a, with a total mass greater than 30 mg/dL is considered elevated with a corresponding Lp(a) cholesterol cut off at 10 mg/dL. Elevated (moderate) plasma homocysteinemia is also associated with increased risk.

Patient stress, especially with hospitalization, adversely affects plasma lipid concentrations, and a fasting specimen (at 12 to 14 hours) is optimal after a low-fat, low-calorie diet with no alcohol ingestion for 24 hours.

Endocrine Function Assessment

Thyroid

An initial, sensitive, thyroid-stimulating hormone (TSH) determination should suffice when it is within normal limits, i.e., euthyroid, because it is the earliest hormone to change in altered thyroid function, except in the presence of pituitary disease. However, the TSH may be within normal limits in subclinical hypothyroidism and may also be elevated in the presence of thyroid hormone resistance and a pituitary tumor.

A free-thyroxine (FT_4) assay should be determined when the TSH is elevated or depressed. When the TSH is elevated, a depressed-thyroxine (T_4) or free-thyroxine (FT_4) value is consistent with hypothyroidism. A depressed TSH with an elevated FT_4 should confirm a diagnosis of hyperthyroidism. Incipient (early) hyperthyroidism can be identified through its association with a normal FT_4 and an elevated FT_3 (T_3 thyrotoxicosis is rare). Nonthyroidal illness and drugs are reflected in a patient with decreased TSH and decreased FT_4.

There are several other causes of increased serum thyroxine (T_4) (Table 12–14) and abnormalities in protein-binding capacity (Table 12–15). Various diseases also reflect changes in thyroid function (Table 12–16).

Cushing Syndrome

Cushing syndrome diagnosis in a patient with central obesity, facial plethora, purple striae, and proximal muscle weakness or unexplained osteoporosis is best accomplished with two 24-hour urinary free-cortisol assays. Alcoholic patients should abstain from drinking for at least a month before urine collection. The 1-mg overnight dexamethasone-suppression test is most useful in patients with equivocal urinary free-cortisol determinations (Table 12–17). False-positive results may be caused by obesity, stress, and psychiatric illness in the presence of elevated plasma cortisol-binding globulin, and chronic renal failure. Liver failure patients may also have false-negative test results.

The paired measurement of cortisol and ACTH should delineate whether the Cushing disease is ACTH independent (adrenocortical lesion) or ACTH dependent. Low-dose and high-dose dexamethasone-suppression tests will demonstrate a low concentration in patients with pituitary-dependent

Table 12–14 □ SOME CAUSES OF INCREASED SERUM T$_4$

Cause	Comment
Increased serum-binding proteins	See Table 12–15
Isolated hyperthyroxinemia	Some patients with nonthyroidal illness ($\uparrow$T$_4$ but T$_3$ not increased)
Familial dysalbuminemic hyperthyroxinemia	Increased affinity of albumin for T$_4$
Familial euthyroid thyroxine excess	Increased affinity of thyroxine-binding prealbumin (TBPA) for T$_4$
Psychiatric disease	? Mechanism
Target organ resistance (a) familial (Refetoff), (b) acquired	Intracellular resistance to thyroid hormone
Other syndromes: (for example, decreased peripheral T$_3$ production)	(Miscellaneous: ? inhibition of T$_4$ transport into tissues or reduced T$_4$ to T$_3$ conversion)
Spurious	Circulating antibody to T$_4$
Drugs (excluding those that $\uparrow$ thyroxine-binding globulin [TBG]); amiodarone,* amphetamine, heparin, heroin, iodine-containing radiocontrast media,* propranolol*	

From Henry JB: Clinical Diagnosis and Management by Laboratory Methods, 19th ed. Philadelphia, WB Saunders Co, 1996, p 336.
*Indicates those drugs that block T$_4$ to T$_3$ conversion.

Cushing syndrome, whereas adrenocortical neoplasms or ectopic ACTH secretions will display minimal suppression (Fig. 12–8).

Catecholamine, Metanephrines, and Vanillylmandelic Acid

Catecholamine-secreting tumors arising from chromaffin cells of the adrenal medulla (pheochromocytoma) and from paragangliomas may be diagnosed by elimination of interfering medications with a timed urine collection concurrent with a hypertensive clinical spell (10- to 60-minute duration) including headache, palpitations, anxiety, tremor, diaphoreses, and chest pain. Concurrent measurements of urinary catecholamines, metanephrines, and vanillylmandelic acid assays should expedite the evaluation if not with a clinical-spell urine specimen then with an appropriate 24-hour urine collection specimen.

Primary aldosteronism is associated with suppressed plasma renin activity (PRA) and increased aldosterone excretion

Table 12–15 □ SOME CAUSES OF ABNORMALITIES IN PROTEIN-BINDING CAPACITY

	Increased Binding Capacity	Decreased Binding Capacity
Thyroxine-binding globulin (TBG)	Acute intermittent porphyria Estrogens Genetic Hepatic disease Hypothyroidism Newborn infants Oral contraceptives Perphenazine Pregnancy	Active acromegaly Androgens Genetic Hepatic disease Nephrotic syndrome Phenytoin Prednisone Severe illness or surgical stress Thyrotoxicosis
Thyroxine-binding prealbumin (TBPA)	Active acromegaly Androgens Prednisone	Nephrotic syndrome Salicylates Severe illness or surgical stress Thyrotoxicosis

From Henry JB: Clinical Diagnosis and Management by Laboratory Methods, 19th ed. Philadelphia, WB Saunders Co, 1996, p 336.

Table 12–16 □ CHANGES IN THYROID FUNCTION TESTS WITH VARIOUS DISEASE STATES

	TSH	T_4	FT_4	T_3
Hyperthyroidism	↓	↑	↑	↑
T_3 toxicosis	nl/↑			↑
Factitious (T_3)	↓	↓	↓	↑
Factitious (T_4)	↓	↑	↑	↑
Hypothyroidism, first degree	↑	↓	↓	nl/↓
Second-degree pituitary/hypothalamic	↑	↓	↓	↓
Second-degree selective deficiency	nl	↓	↓	↓
Nonthyroidal illness	↓/nl	↓/nl/↑	nl	↓
Psychiatric NTI		↑	↑	↑
Peripheral hormone resistance	nl	↑	↑	↑
Familial dysalbuminemic hyperthyroxinemia (FDH)	nl	↑	nl	nl
TBG deficiency	nl	↓	nl	↓
FDH + TBG deficiency	nl	nl	nl	↓
HIV+	nl	nl	nl	nl
AIDS with secondary infection	nl	nl	nl	↓

From Henry JB: Clinical Diagnosis and Management by Laboratory Methods, 19th ed. Philadelphia, WB Saunders Co, 1996, p 336.
nl = Normal.

Table 12–17 □ SERUM CORTICOSTEROID RESPONSES TO DIAGNOSTIC MANEUVERS DESIGNED TO DEMONSTRATE NONAUTONOMY OR AUTONOMY OF ADRENAL FUNCTION

Condition	Basal (0800-Hour)	Circadian Variation	0800-Hour Response to Dexamethasone (1 mg at 2300 hours)	Response to Aqueous Pitressin (10 Units IM)	Response to Cosyntropin	0800-Hour Plasma ACTH
			Serum Cortisol Concentrations			
Normal	10–25 μg/dL (276–690 nmol/L)	A.M. greater than P.M.	<6 μg/dL (166 nmol/L)	≥15 μg/dL (414 nmol/L) increase above baseline	Doubling of baseline value	20–100 pg/mL (4.4–22 pmol/L)
Adrenal hyperplasia	Normal or increased	Absent	>6 μg/dL (166 nmol/L)	Increased	Increased	Normal or increased
Adrenal adenoma	Normal or increased	Absent	>6 μg/dL (166 nmol/L)	Absent	None or normal	Decreased
Adrenal carcinoma	Increased	Absent	>6 μg/dL (166 nmol/L)	Absent	None	Decreased
Pituitary tumor	Increased	Absent	>6 μg/dL (166 nmol/L)	Absent	None to slight	Markedly increased
Ectopic ACTH syndrome	Increased	Absent	>6 μg/dL (166 nmol/L)	Absent	Usually none	Markedly increased

Modified from Krieger DT: Diagnosis and management of Cushing's syndrome. Syllabus, 28th Postgraduate Assembly of the Endocrine Society. Bethesda, MD, 1976.

Chemistry and Immunology **221**

Synthesis and metabolism of adrenal steroids

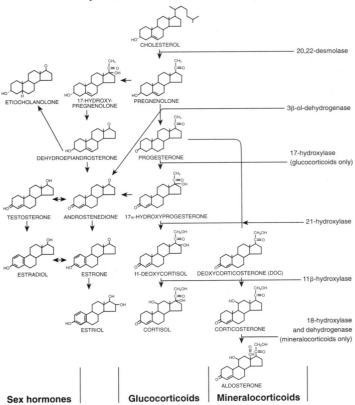

Figure 12–8 □ Simplified pathways of adrenocortical hormone synthesis and metabolism. (From Henry JB: Clinical Diagnosis and Management by Laboratory Methods, 19th ed. Philadelphia, WB Saunders Co, 1996, p 348.)

(plasma aldosterone concentration, or PAC) in patients with hypertension and hypokalemia, though normokalemia may be present in some subtypes. Paired measurements of PRA and PAC are best for screening. A positive screen is followed by PAC measurement after 3 days of salt loading with potassium supplementation. In a 24-hour urine specimen on the third day for aldosterone assay and sodium and potassium measurements, a urinary aldosterone measurement greater than 12 mg/24-hour urine and urinary sodium greater than 200 mEq/L (with adequate sodium load) are consistent with hyperaldosteronism.

Table 12–18 □ **SOME CAUSES OF HYPERTENSION ASSOCIATED WITH LOW LEVELS OF PLASMA RENIN**

"Primary" excess of mineralocorticoids
  Primary aldosteronism
  Pseudoprimary (idiopathic) aldosteronism
  Glucocorticoid-suppressible aldosteronism
  11-Deoxycorticosterone excess
  18-Hydroxy-11-deoxycorticosterone excess
  Adrenal carcinoma (mineralocorticoid excess)
"Secondary" excess of mineralocorticoids
  Licorice ingestion
  Excess unsupervised sodium intake
  Low renin, low aldosterone syndrome
  1. Long-standing essential hypertension
  2. Diabetes mellitus

From Henry JB: Clinical Diagnosis and Management by Laboratory Methods, 19th ed. Philadelphia, WB Saunders Co, 1996, p 358.

Hypertension and Plasma Renin

Several causes of hypertension are associated with low levels of plasma renin (Table 12–18) and high levels of plasma renin (Table 12–19).

Plasma Aldosterone Concentration (PAC) and Plasma Renin Activity (PRA)

Both assays are useful in patients with hypertension and hypokalemia. The PAC-to-PRA ratio may allow identification of other causes of hypertension and hypokalemia, as follows:

↑PRA (ng/mL/h)	↓PRA (ng/mL/h)
↑PAC (ng/dL)	↓PAC (ng/dL)
PAC/PRA ratio ≤10	
Seek causes of aldosteronism:	Evaluate
Coarctation of the aorta	Altered aldosterone metabolism
Diuretic use	Congenital adrenal hyperplasia
Malignant-phase hypertension	Cushing syndrome
Renin-secreting tumor	Deoxycorticosterone-producing tumor
Renovascular hypertension	Exogenous mineralocorticoid
	11β-hydroxysteroid dehydrogenase deficiency
	Liddle syndrome

A PAC/PRA ratio >20 and a PAC ≥20 ng/dL should prompt investigation for primary aldosteronism.

Table 12–19 □ SOME CAUSES OF HYPERTENSION ASSOCIATED WITH HIGH LEVELS OF PLASMA RENIN

Renin-secreting tumor
Malignant accelerated hypertension
Renovascular hypertension
   Major arterial lesions
   Segmental lesions
Chronic renal failure
   End stage
   Transplant rejection
Cushing's syndrome
Iatrogenic
   Volume-depleting agents
   Vasodilating agents
   Glucocorticoids
   Estrogens

From Henry JB: Clinical Diagnosis and Management by Laboratory Methods, 19th ed. Philadelphia, WB Saunders Co, 1996, p 357.

Prolactin

The causes of elevated serum prolactin levels are shown in Table 12–20.

Antidiuretic Hormone/Water Homeostasis

Antidiuretic hormone (ADH) excess or deficiency are manifested as the syndrome of inappropriate ADH secretion (SIADH) and diabetes insipidus (DI) respectively. Differential diagnosis of

Table 12–20 CAUSES OF ELEVATED SERUM PROLACTIN LEVELS

Physiologic	Pathologic	Iatrogenic (Medications)
Exercise	Acromegaly	Metoclopramide
Neonate	Cirrhosis (alcoholic)	Methyldopa
Nursing	Empty sella syndrome	Reserpine
Pregnancy	Hypothalamic lesions	Verapamil
Sleep	Primary hypothyroidism	TRH
Stress	Nelson's syndrome	Cimetidine (intravenous)
Dietary protein	Neurogenic	Estrogens
Hypoglycemia	Pituitary prolactinomas	Opioid narcotics
	Pituitary stalk lesions	Chlorpromazine
	Renal failure	Haloperidol
	VIPoma	Serotonin-reuptake inhibitors
	Generalized seizures	

From Henry JB: Clinical Diagnosis and Management by Laboratory Methods, 19th ed. Philadelphia, WB Saunders Co, 1996, p 329.
TRH = Thyrotropin-releasing hormone.

Table 12–21 □ TESTS IN THE DIFFERENTIAL DIAGNOSIS OF DISORDERS OF WATER HOMEOSTASIS

Disorder	Baseline			After 12-Hour Fluid Restriction			
	Serum Na+ and Osm	Urine Na+ and Osm	Serum ADH	Serum Na+ and Osm	Urine Na+ and Osm	Serum ADH	Urine Osm Post AVP Challenge
Normal Control	N	N	N	N	High	High	Same
SIADH	Low	N-High	High	Low-N	High	High	Same
Neurogenic DI	N-High	Low	Low	High	Low-N	Low	Increased
Nephrogenic DI	N-High	Low	N-High	High	Low-N	High	Same
Psychogenic Polydipsia	Low-N	Low	Low	N	N-High	N-High	Same

From Henry JB: Clinical Diagnosis and Management by Laboratory Methods, 19th ed. Philadelphia, WB Saunders Co, 1996, p 332.
SIADH = Syndrome of inappropriate antidiuretic hormone secretion; DI = diabetes insipidus; Osm = osmolality; ADH = antidiuretic hormone; AVP = arginine vasopressin; N = normal.

these two conditions by laboratory determinations is shown in Table 12–21.

Gonadotropins

Gonadotropin-releasing hormone (GnRH) controls the secretion of the gonadotropins (luteinizing hormone, LH; follicle-stimulating hormone, FSH) from the anterior pituitary same population of cells. The older name for GnRH is luteinizing-releasing hormone (LRH).

Abnormalities in gonadotropin concentrations may reflect hypergonadotropism or hypogonadotropism (low GnRH or decreased or no pulse frequency) as common causes of secondary amenorrhea and also delayed menarche. Hypergonadism may result in precocious puberty. Table 12–22 shows basal hormone blood levels in disorders of the hypothalamic-pituitary-gonadal axis in men, with the understanding that acute illness affects this axis. LH, FSH, and testosterone levels decrease in proportion to the severity of disease or illness in men and postmenopausal women with a gradual rebound or return to normal levels as the disease subsides and health is regained.

Polycystic ovary disease is the most common cause of androgen-dependent hirsutism (Table 12–23). In these patients free testosterone (preferable to serum total testosterone) is usually elevated.

Sex hormone-binding globulin (SHBG) as a carrier protein that binds estradiol, estriol, estrone, and also testosterone is an important consideration in total serum sex hormone assays versus free-hormone assays.

■ VIRAL HEPATITIS TESTING AND SEROLOGY

Diagnosis of acute hepatitis in a jaundiced patient involves a battery of tests in the clinical pathology laboratory. These include liver-function tests and serologic tests for viral cause. Tests of liver function are often offered as organ/disease panels (Table 12–5) and serve to evaluate metabolic and synthetic functions of the liver. Serum aminotransferase levels are typically elevated, whereas other enzyme levels may be elevated to a lesser degree. Prolongation of the prothrombin time (PT) is a good indicator of the severity of liver injury. (See the discussion of hepatic function, p. 209.)

At least six different hepatitis viruses are known (hepatitis A, B, C, D, E, G viruses) (Table 12–24). Many other viruses can cause hepatitis, and numerous nonviral causes of acute hepatitis exist. In the investigation of acute hepatitis, a battery of serologic tests should be used to detect the commonly implicated viral agents (Table 12–25). The most common agents in the United States are hepatitis B, C, and A viruses. Therefore, initial testing should include the following:

- Anti-hepatitis A virus (anti-HAV) IgM (positive in recent hepatitis A infection)

Table 12–22 □ BASAL HORMONE LEVELS IN DISORDERS OF THE HYPOTHALAMIC-PITUITARY-GONADAL AXIS IN MEN

Diagnosis	LH	FSH	Testosterone	Estradiol
Hypothalamus and pituitary (hypogonadotropic syndromes)				
Hypopituitarism	↓ or N*	↓ or N	↓ or N	↓ or N
Kallmann syndrome	↓ or N	↓ or N	↓ or N	↓ or N
Isolated gonadotropin deficiency	↓ or N	↓ or N	↓ or N	↓ or N
Simple delayed puberty	↓ or N	↓ or N	↓	↓
Gonad (hypergonadotropic syndromes)				
Primary testicular failure	↑↑	↑↑	↓↓	↓ or N
Anorchism	↑↑	↑↑	↓↓	↓ or N
Cryptorchidism	N or ↑	N or ↑	N	N
Azoospermia and oligospermia	N	N or ↑	N	N
Varicocele	N	N or ↑	N	N or ↑
Klinefelter's syndrome	↑ or N	↑	↓ or N	N or ↑
Complete testicular feminization syndrome	↑	↑ or N	N or ↑	↑
Precocious puberty				
Idiopathic or central nervous system lesion	↑↑	↑↑	↑↑	↑ or N
Adrenal tumors or congenital adrenal hyperplasia	↓	↓	↑↑	↑ or N

Modified from Marshall JC: Clin Endocrinol Metab 1975; 4:545. (c) The Endocrine Soc.
*Normal represented by N, increases and decreases by arrows.

Table 12–23 □ CAUSES OF ANDROGEN-DEPENDENT HIRSUTISM

Ovarian causes

Neoplastic
    Sertoli-Leydig cell tumors (arrhenoblastoma)
    Granulosa-stromal cell tumors
    Gonadoblastoma
    Lipoid cell tumor
Non-neoplastic
    Polycystic ovarian disease
    Hyperthecosis
    Idiopathic hirsutism

Adrenal abnormalities

Neoplastic
    Adrenocortical carcinoma
    Virilizing adrenal adenoma
Non-neoplastic
    Congenital adrenal hyperplasia
        21-Hydroxylase deficiency
        11-Hydroxylase deficiency
    Cushing's disease
Medications
    Androgens (danazol, fluoxymesterone [Halotestin])
    19-Nortestosterone derivatives

From Henry JB: Clinical Diagnosis and Management by Laboratory Methods, 19th ed. Philadelphia, WB Saunders Co, 1996, p 366.

- Hepatitis B surface antigen (HBsAg) (positive in acute or chronic hepatitis B)
- Anti-hepatitis B core antigen (anti-HBc) (positive in current or past hepatitis B infection)
- Anti-hepatitis C virus (anti-HCV) (may be negative in early infection)

If there is a history of travel, anti-hepatitis E virus (anti-HEV) antibody should be measured. If clinical suspicion of hepatitis C persists, HCV-RNA can be measured by reference laboratories (anti-HCV may appear late). Since hepatitis D virus infection occurs only in the presence of hepatitis B, antibodies to hepatitis D virus are useful in evaluating exacerbations in patients with known HBV infection.

If serologic tests for hepatitis viruses are negative, other etiologic agents should be considered, including Epstein-Barr virus, cytomegalovirus, drug-induced hepatitis, autoimmune hepatitis, biliary obstruction, etc.

Text continued on page 232

Table 12–24 □ CLINICAL FEATURES OF HEPATITIS VIRUS INFECTIONS

	Hepatitis A	Hepatitis B	Hepatitis C	Hepatitis D	Hepatitis E
Classification	Picornaviridae (enterovirus 72)	Hepadnaviridae	Flaviviridae	(Satellite)	(Calicivirus)
Genotype(s)	One	At least 8	At least 6	One	One
Mean incubation time (range)	4 weeks (10–50 days)	12 weeks (14–180 days)	8 weeks (1–24 days)	3–13 weeks	6 weeks (14–63 days)
Chronicity	No	5–10% infected adults, 25–50% children, 70–90% infants	>60 (20% develop cirrhosis)	10–15%	No
Risk of hepatocellular carcinoma	No	Yes, high association	Yes, low association	?	No
Mortality, acute hepatitis	About 0.6%	About 1.4%	1–2%	Up to 30%	1–2%; up to 20% in pregnant women

From Henry JB: Clinical Diagnosis and Management by Laboratory Methods, 19th ed. Philadelphia, WB Saunders Co, 1996, p 1108.

Table 12–25 □ SEROLOGIC MARKERS IN THE DIAGNOSIS OF HEPATITIS

	IgM anti-HAV	Anti-HAV	HBsAg	Anti-HBs	IgM anti-HBc	Anti-HBc	HBeAg	Anti-HBe	HBV-DNA	Anti-HCV	Anti-HDV	Anti-HEV
Acute Infection												
HAV	+	+										
HBV												
Early			+	–	+	+	+	–	–			
Window			–	–	+	+	+/–	–	–			
Resolving			–	+	–	+	+	+	–			
HCV										+/–		
HDV												
Coinfection			+/–	–	+	+	–	–	+		+	
Superinfection			+/–	–	–	+	+/–	–/+	+/–		+	
HEV												+
Chronic Infection												
HBV												
Nonreplicating			+	–	–	+	–	+	–			
Replicating			+	–	–	+	+	–	+			
Reactivation			+	–	+	+	+	–	+			
HCV										+		
HDV			+	–	–	+	–/+	+/–	–/+		+	

Table continued on following page

Table 12–25 □ SEROLOGIC MARKERS IN THE DIAGNOSIS OF HEPATITIS *Continued*

	IgM anti-HAV	Anti-HAV	HBsAg	Anti-HBs	IgM anti-HBc	Anti-HBc	HBeAg	Anti-HBe	HBV-DNA	Anti-HCV	Anti-HDV	Anti-HEV
Past Infection												
HAV	–	+										
HBV			–	+	–	+	–	+	–			
HCV										+		
HDV			–	+/–	–	+	–	+	–		+	
HEV												+

Modified from Biesemier KW, Parks D, Gertis C, et al: Bull Lab Med 1994; 134.
  HDV = hepatitis D virus; HEV = hepatitis E virus; HBs = hepatitis B surface antigen; HBe = hepatitis E antigen; HBc = hepatitis B core antigen; + = positive; – = negative.

STATE UNIVERSITY OF NEW YORK
Health Science Center at Syracuse
John Doe   Transplant Surgeon   Dr.
750 E. Adams St., Syracuse, NY

123456   CLINICAL PATHOLOGY - SPECIAL

DATE: 11/29/99   No. 12345

Renal Transplant Candidate

Date of Sample: 1/1/1999
Date of Testing: 1/1/1999

HISTOCOMPATIBILITY ANTIGEN TYPING REPORT

NAME	RELATIONSHIP	HLA-A	HLA-B	HLA-C	HLA-DR	ABO
Doe, John		A1,A2	B8,B62		DR3,9	A
Doe, James	Sibling	A1,A32	B8,B27		DR15,3	A
	Lymphocytotoxic Antibody:			Negative		
	Lymphocytotoxic Crossmatch:					
	T-Cell:			Negative		
	B-Cell:			Negative		

Previous Transplant (6/1/1989)
Cadaver Donor URS009: HLA: A2, A11 B14,B35   DR7,8   A

ABO typing(s) were performed by the Blood Bank, University Hospital,
Syracuse, New York.

Comments: The patient is a 21 y/o male with ESRD secondary to obstructive
uropathy and ureteral reflux since 1985, on dialysis since 1988. S/p cadaveric
renal transplant in 1989, which functioned until return to dialysis in 1998. He
is now on peritoneal dialysis pending his scheduled living donor transplant
on 1/2/1999. He is a one-haplotype match with his brother. They are ABO
compatible. T- and B-cell crossmatches employing current as well as historical
sera were negative. His brother does not share any mismatched antigens
with the patient's previous transplant donor. The patient's serum was screened
by a solid-phase Enzyme Immunosorbent Assay (ELISA) used to detect IgG
antibodies to HLA Class I antigens. No cytotoxic antibody was detected.

John Bernard Henry, MD
Director/Transfusion Medicine

Figure 12–9 □ Solid organ transplantation patient report.

Hepatitides B, C, D, and G can lead to chronic infection. Evaluation of chronic hepatitis includes tests for HBsAg, anti-HCV, and anti-HDV. The presence of HBeAg indicates active replication, but HBeAg is replaced by anti-HBe in nonreplicating chronic carriers.

■ HIV CONFIDENTIALITY ISSUES

HIV testing is performed by many laboratories, and laws regarding confidentiality of data must be observed. In New York State, HIV testing may be performed only after an informed written consent (except when the patient's identification is not known or for organ or tissue transplantation purposes) is obtained. The laboratory information system should have adequate safeguards to prevent unauthorized persons from gaining access to HIV-related data, and usually the number of persons with such access should be kept to a minimum. Release of HIV information by phone or facsimile is prohibited. Results are released only by mail to the ordering physician and are clearly marked confidential.

■ TESTING FOR ORGAN OR TISSUE TRANSPLANTATION

A standard protocol should be available for performing tests required for organ or tissue transplantation. Organs or tissues for transplantation often become available during off hours. Although the pathologist provides an interpretation of high-resolution DNA typing with other technologists, oversight and coordination also are important. Some common tests performed for release of organs for transplantation include CMV and EBV antibodies, rapid plasma reagin test for syphilis, HIV 1 and 2 antibodies, hepatitis B surface antigen, human T-cell leukemia/lymphoma virus (HTLV) 1 and 2 antibodies, hepatitis C antibody, hepatitis B core antibody, and hepatitis B surface antibody. Additionally the tissue-typing laboratory is involved in performing HLA typing on the donor or donors and crossmatches for a possible solid-organ recipient with their historic sera including the highest-percentage reaction antibody (PRA). Final review of crossmatches, most likely recipient optimal match, and sign-off with a transplant surgeon usually complete the process (Fig. 12–9).

MICROSCOPY

Special competency in both light microscopy and phase microscopy, coupled with an in-depth knowledge of urine and other body fluids, provide the on-call resident with a solid foundation to make important and continuing contributions to patient care through this laboratory section.

An ability to critically analyze and evaluate the examination of urine, cerebrospinal fluid (CSF), synovial fluid, and peritoneal, pleural, and other fluids including unknown specimens from any body or portion site or source is central to an effective role. Just as in other laboratory sections, there is no substitute for first-hand knowledge, derived from training, reading, and experience at the bench and the bedside or clinic, with patients and their personal physicians. Since this will not likely be accomplished during time allocated to a resident's rotation, there is limited exposure to less commonly encountered specimens, diseases, and reports of results. It is incumbent, therefore, on the resident and technical staff in Microscopy to develop a system for retention or retrieval, with appropriate transportation and storage for preservation within the laboratory, of interesting, significant specimens or constituents in urine and other body fluids from the daily work load. Residents not on assignment in Microscopy can then avail themselves of an opportunity at a mutually convenient time (to staff and resident) to review and examine some of the most interesting body fluids and their constituents with related physical, chemical, and bacteriologic analyses, along with relevant clinical and laboratory information. Access to patients and clinical colleagues caring for such patients then can provide both a learning and service experience and over time a wealth of knowledge and understanding of disease not available otherwise. Like so many other things, "If you don't use it, you will lose it." There is no substitute for confidence as well as competence in identification of formed elements in urine, crystals, and other constituents in all body fluids; they may yield important and uniquely available diagnostic and clinical management information. This requires a sustained effort over a long time, i.e., years, to accomplish.

◼ ROLE OF RESIDENT ON CALL

- Identify or confirm presence of urinary true blood casts, red blood cell (RBC) casts, and renal tubular epithelial casts observed in patients with acute renal failure (ARF); ARF is encountered in up to 30% of hospitalized patients, especially in critical care units.
- Correlate findings with patient's disease or illness and the cause of renal failure (Table 13–1).
- When clinical suspicion is high and urine findings do not correlate, a fresh specimen should be collected to verify acid pH with an optimal specific gravity ~1.018 or higher; prompt examination is essential (Table 13–2).
- Identify or confirm presence of leukocyte (WBC) casts, diagnostic of acute pyelonephritis in a comparable manner. Recognize other casts (Table 13–3).
- Check patients whose urine has a dark brown or black color or appearance and differentiate its cause (Table 13–4). Also consider, (1) if acid pH, test for melanogens to confirm melanogenuria, which may occur in patients with metastatic malignant melanoma, (2) if alkaline pH, alkaptonuria or ochronosis should be suspected; confirm with identification of homogentisic acid, and (3) presence of blood as red blood cells in concentrated (~1.015 specific gravity or higher) or as hemoglobin in dilute or hypotonic (1.010 or less) acid urine with delineation of hemoglobinuria and hematuria. Rule out presence of *myoglobin* to confirm rhabdomyolysis (see Table 13–4).
- Verify an optimal fresh urine collection as acid pH (6.0 or less) and concentrated (specific gravity of 1.015 or higher), needed for casts to be observed, and resolve discrepancies in urinalysis results or clinical correlation called to your attention.
- Be suspicious when examining an alkaline urine specimen and its results interpretation. Urea, $C \overset{\diagup NH_2}{\underset{\diagdown NH_2}{=} O}$, in the presence of urease-splitting bacteria, releases ammonium ions, which react with water to form ammonium hydroxide and an alkaline urine.
- An alkaline urine pH of 7.0 or greater signifies most frequently three possibilities that must be checked to establish quality and nature of urine specimen:
  - Old urine (several hours) stored at room temperature—unacceptable
  - Postprandial (alkaline tide) urine collection—limited if any value for detection of urinary casts and cells
  - Urinary tract infection and most likely bacterial cause of *Proteus* or *Pseudomonas* to a lesser extent

- Review, confirm, and correlate clinically all abnormal CSF and other body fluid cell counts (Table 13–5).
- Identify and differentiate crystals in synovial fluid, i.e., pyrophosphate observed in pseudogout and uric acid crystals of gout.

Table 13–1 □ ACUTE RENAL FAILURE: ETIOLOGY AND CORRELATIONS

Pre-renal Azotemia (~70%)

Volume depletion or decreased effective circulatory volume
U/A: hyaline casts, SG > 1.018
Response to restoration of renal perfusion

Intrinsic Renal Azotemia (~25%)

Large Vessel Causes

Renal Artery Thrombosis
Diagnosis: atrial fibrillation, nausea/vomiting, flank/abdominal pain
U/A: mild proteinuria, occasional red blood cells

Atheroembolism
Recent procedure, vasculopathy, livedo reticularis, retinal plaques
U/A: Normal $+/-$ eosinophils
Other: eosinophilia, low C3/C4

Renal Vein Thrombosis
Nephrotic or pulmonary embolus, flank pain
U/A: proteinuria, hematuria

Diseases of Small Vessels and Glomeruli

Glomerulitis/Vasculitis
Multisystem, lung hemorrhage, rash, skin ulcer, arthralgias
U/A: red blood cell casts, dysmorphic red blood cells, proteinuria
Studies: C3, ANCA, anti-GBM, ANA, anti-DNA, ASO, cryoglobulins, hepatic serologic assays, renal biopsy

Hemolytic Uremic Syndrome and Thrombotic Thrombocytopenic Purpura
GI infection, purpura, fever, central nervous system symptoms, cyclosporin A
U/A: normal, mild red blood cells/proteinuria, rare red blood cells/granular casts
Studies: microangiopathic hemolytic anemia, lactate dehydrogenase ↑, platelets ↓, microangiopathic peripheral blood smear

Malignant Hypertension
Papilledema, congestive heart failure, retinopathy, neurologic symptoms
U/A: red blood cells, red blood cell casts, proteinuria
Studies: left ventricular hypertrophy, improves with early blood pressure control

KEY: ANA = antinuclear antibody; ANCA = antineutrophil cytoplasmic antibody; ASO = antistreptolysin O; CRF = chronic renal failure; GBM = glomerular basement membrane; SG = specific gravity; U/A = Urinalysis.

Table continued on following page

Table 13–1 □ **ACUTE RENAL FAILURE:**
ETIOLOGY AND CORRELATIONS *Continued*

Acute Tubular Necrosis

Ischemia
Recent hemorrhage, hypotension, major surgery, burns
U/A: muddy brown granular casts, renal tubular epithelial cells
Studies: biopsy

Exogenous Toxins
Contrasts, abdominal examination, anti-cancer agents often with
   hypovolemia/sepsis/CRF
U/A: muddy brown granular casts, renal tubular epithelial cells
Studies: biopsy

Endogenous Toxins
Rhabdomyolysis (seizures, ethanol, trauma), hemolysis, tumorolysis,
   myeloma, ethylene glycol
U/A: heme (+), urate crystals, dipstick (−) protein, oxalate crystals
Studies: K, phosphorus, Ca, urine myoglobin, creatine kinase, uric acid,
   serum protein electrophoresis/urine protein electrophoresis, toxicology,
   osmolality gap, acidosis

Acute Tubulointerstitial Diseases

Allergic Interstitial Nephritis
New drug, fever, rash, arthralgias
U/A: white blood cells, white blood cell casts, red blood cells, proteinuria,
   eosinophils
Studies: eosinophilia, skin biopsy, renal biopsy

Acute Bilateral Pyelonephritis
Flank pain and tenderness, toxic, female
U/A: white blood cells, white blood cell casts, proteinuria, bacteria, red
   blood cells
Studies: urine and blood cultures

Post-renal Azotemia (~5%)

Abdominal or flank pain, palpable bladder, nodular prostatic hyperplasia
U/A: normal, occasional red blood cells
Studies: kidney urinary bladder roentgenogram, ultrasonogram,
   intravenous pyelogram, computerized tomography

- Confirm or correlate chylous effusion in pleural and peritoneal
  fluids, which may be attributed to thoracic duct obstruction
  (Table 13–6).
- Follow up abnormal measurements of urine protein reflecting
  massive proteinuria, with particular attention to a sudden increase when greater than a range of 5 to 10 g present in a total
  Text continued on page 243

Table 13-2 □ VARIOUS URINARY SYSTEM DISEASES AND CORRESPONDING URINALYSIS ABNORMALITIES

Diseases	Macroscopic Urinalysis	Microscopic Urinalysis
Acute glomerulonephritis	Gross hematuria "Smoky" turbidity Proteinuria	Erythrocyte and blood casts Epithelial casts Hyaline and granular casts Waxy casts Neutrophils Erythrocytes
Chronic glomerulonephritis	Hematuria Proteinuria	Granular and waxy casts Occasional blood casts Erythrocytes Leukocytes Epithelial casts Lipid droplets
Acute pyelonephritis	Turbid Occasional odor Occasional proteinuria	Numerous neutrophils (many in clumps) Few lymphocytes and histiocytes Leukocyte casts Epithelial casts Renal epithelial cells Erythrocytes Granular and waxy casts Bacteria

Table continued on following page

Table 13-2 □ VARIOUS URINARY SYSTEM DISEASES AND CORRESPONDING URINALYSIS ABNORMALITIES *Continued*

Diseases	Macroscopic Urinalysis	Microscopic Urinalysis
Chronic pyelonephritis	Occasional proteinuria	Leukocytes Broad waxy casts Granular and epithelial casts Occasional leukocyte cast Bacteria Erythrocytes
Nephrotic syndrome	Proteinuria Fat droplets	Fatty and waxy casts Cellular and granular casts Oval fat bodies or vacuolated renal epithelial cells occurring singly or as cellular clusters
Acute tubular necrosis	Hematuria Occasional proteinuria	Necrotic or degenerated renal epithelial cells Neutrophils and erythrocytes Granular and epithelial casts Waxy casts Broad casts Epithelial tissue fragments
Cystitis	Hematuria	Numerous leukocytes Erythrocytes Transitional epithelial cells occurring singly or as fragments Histiocytes and giant cells Bacteria Absence of casts

Dysuria-pyuria syndrome	Slightly turbid	Numerous leukocytes, bacteria Erythrocytes No casts
Acute renal allograft rejection (lower nephrosis)	Hematuria Occasional proteinuria	Renal epithelial cells Lymphocytes and plasma cells Neutrophils Renal epithelial casts Renal epithelial fragments Granular, bloody, and waxy casts
Urinary tract neoplasia	Hematuria	Atypical mononuclear cells with enlarged, irregular hyperchromatic nuclei and sometimes containing prominent nucleoli that occur singly or as tissue fragments Neutrophils Erythrocytes Transitional epithelial cells
Viral infection	Hematuria Occasional proteinuria	Enlarged mononuclear cells or multinucleated cells with prominent intranuclear or cytoplasmic inclusions Neutrophils Lymphocytes and plasma cells Erythrocytes

From Henry JB: Clinical Diagnosis and Management by Laboratory Methods, 19th ed. Philadelphia, WB Saunders Co, 1996, p 439.

Table 13–3 □ CLASSIFICATION OF CASTS

Matrix
   Hyaline—variable size
   Waxy—often broad in use
Inclusions
   Granules—proteins, cell debris
   Fat globules—triglycerides, cholesterol esters
   Hemosiderin granules
   Crystals—uncommon
   Melanin granules—rare
Pigments
   Hemoglobin, myoglobin, bilirubin, drugs
Cells
   Erythrocytes and red blood cell remnants
   Leukocytes—neutrophils, lymphocytes, monocytes, and histiocytes
   Renal tubular epithelial cells
   Mixed cells—erythrocytes, neutrophils, and renal tubular cells
   Bacteria

From Henry JB: Clinical Diagnosis and Management by Laboratory Methods, 19th ed. Philadelphia, WB Saunders Co, 1996, p 441.

Table 13–4 □ DIFFERENTIATION OF HEMATURIA, HEMOGLOBINURIA, AND MYOGLOBINURIA

Condition	Plasma Findings	Urine Findings

Hematuria	Color—normal	Color—normal, smoky, pink, red, brown
		Erythrocytes—many
		  Renal—red blood cell casts
		  Protein—significant increase
		  Lower urinary tract—no casts
		  Protein—present or absent

Hemoglobinuria	Color—pink (early) Haptoglobin—low	Color—pink, red, brown Erythrocytes—occasional Pigment casts—occasional Protein—present or absent Hemosiderin—late
Myoglobinuria	Color—normal Haptoglobin—normal Creatine kinase—significant increase Aldolase—increased	Color—red, brown Erythrocytes—occasional Dense brown casts—occasional Protein—present or absent

From Henry JB: Clinical Diagnosis and Management by Laboratory Methods, 19th ed. Philadelphia, WB Saunders Co, 1996, p 430.

Table 13-5 □ CEREBROSPINAL FLUID FINDINGS IN MENINGITIS

Meningitis	Opening Pressure	Leukocytes/μL	Protein (mg/dL)	Glucose (mg/dL)*	Comments
Acute bacterial	Usually increased	1000–10,000 or more; occasionally <100 PMNs	Most 100–500	Usually <40	Partially treated cases may convert to lymphocytosis; most retain the other abnormalities
Viral	Normal to moderate increase	5–300; some >1000; lymphocytes and PMNs may predominate in first 24–36 hr	Normal to mildly increased (most <100)	Normal	Reduced glucose seen in 25% of cases of mumps, some HSV
Fungal	Increased	40–400; lymphocytes or PMNs predominate; eosinophilia may be found in Coccidioides	50–300; average about 100	Decreased	Neutrophilic pleocytosis most common with mycelial fungal forms
Tuberculous	Increased; decreased with spinal block	100–600 up to 1200. Mixed or lymphocytic; PMNs often predominate early	50–300 significant increase with spinal block	Decreased; <45 in many cases	Findings vary depending on clinical stage

Table continued on following page

Table 13–5 □ CEREBROSPINAL FLUID FINDINGS IN MENINGITIS *Continued*

Meningitis	Opening Pressure	Leukocytes/μL	Protein (mg/dL)	Glucose (mg/dL)*	Comments
Acute syphilitic	Increased	Average 500; lymphocytic, rarely neutrophilic	Increased, usually no more than 100	Normal	Up to 15% have normal CSF parameters
Amebic (*Naegleria*)	Increased	Mildly increased to grossly purulent (>20,000); PMNs	Increased, may reach 1000	Normal to decreased	RBCs suggest hemorrhagic brain necrosis
Lyme disease (Stage II findings)	Increased	5–400; lymphocytes predominate	Normal to increased, most <300	Normal to decreased	CSF normal in early infection (Stage I)
Carcinomatous	Normal to increased	0 to hundreds; lymphocytes predominate; variable number of tumor cells may be seen	Usually increased; most <500	Decreased in most cases	Marked neutrophilic pleocytosis may be seen in large necrotic tumors

Modified from Fishman RA: Cerebrospinal Fluid in Diseases of the Nervous System, 2nd ed. Philadelphia, WB Saunders Co, 1992.
*In presence of normal serum levels.

Table 13–6 □ DISTINGUISHING FEATURES IN CHYLOUS AND PSEUDOCHYLOUS EFFUSIONS

	Chylous	Pseudochylous
Onset	Sudden	Gradual
Appearance	Milky-white, or yellow-bloody	Milky or greenish, metallic sheen
Microscopic examination	Lymphocytosis	Mixed cellular reaction, cholesterol crystals
Triglycerides	>110 mg/dL (>1.24 mmol/L)	<50 mg/dL (<0.56 mmol/L)*
Lipoprotein electrophoresis	Chylomicrons present	Chylomicrons absent

Modified from Kjeldsberg CR, Knight JA: Body Fluids: Laboratory Examination of Amniotic, Cerebrospinal, Seminal, Serous and Synovial Fluids, 3rd ed. © American Society of Clinical Pathologists, Chicago, 1993.
*Some pseudochylous effusions have triglyceride levels higher than 110 mg/dL.
Values in parentheses are SI units.

24-hour specimen collection, especially on weekends; these need to be called to the attending physician for patients with nephrotic syndrome and especially preeclampsia/eclampsia, which may herald a significant clinical change, necessitating patient reassessment with a modification in clinical management including hospitalization.
- Review, confirm, and clinically correlate any unusual urinary microscopic findings as well as any unusual body fluid findings (Tables 13–7 and 13–8).
- Evaluate all suspect body fluid slides and unusual urine microscopic preparations for abnormal cells.
- Check all crystal analyses and correlate with other urine findings.
- Differentiate transudate fluid and exudates (Table 13–9).

■ URINE CASTS

Since the identification of urine casts may be crucial in establishing a diagnosis, a brief review follows.

Casts are cylindrical bodies representing an actual cast of the tubular lumen. They may be formed anywhere along the course of the nephron by precipitation of protein or by conglutination of material within the lumen.

The clinical significance of casts is that they are formed within renal parenchyma. They may show or include, within their stroma, red blood cells, epithelial cells, and white blood cells; when such cells are present, it is inferred that they originated within renal substance.

Table 13–7 □ CAUSES OF PERICARDIAL EFFUSIONS

Infection
   Bacterial pericarditis
   Tuberculosis
   Fungal pericarditis
   Viral or mycoplasmal pericarditis
   AIDS-related
Neoplasm
   Metastatic carcinoma
   Lymphoma
Myocardial infarct
Hemorrhage
   Trauma
   Anticoagulant therapy
   Leakage of aortic aneurysm
Metabolic
   Uremia
   Myxedema
Rheumatoid disease
Systemic lupus erythematosus

From Henry JB: Clinical Diagnosis and Management by Laboratory Methods, 19th ed. Philadelphia, WB Saunders Co, 1996, p 476.

Table 13–8 □ CAUSES OF PERITONEAL EFFUSIONS

Transudates (increased hydrostatic pressure or decreased plasma oncotic pressure)
   Congestive heart failure
   Hepatic cirrhosis
   Hypoproteinemia (e.g., nephrotic syndrome)
Exudates (increased capillary permeability or decreased lymphatic resorption)
   Infections
      Tuberculosis
      Primary bacterial peritonitis
      Secondary bacterial peritonitis (e.g., appendicitis)
   Neoplasms
      Hepatoma
      Metastatic carcinoma
      Lymphoma
      Mesothelioma
   Trauma
   Pancreatitis
   Bile peritonitis (e.g., ruptured gallbladder)
Chylous effusion
   Damage or obstruction to thoracic duct (e.g., trauma, lymphoma, carcinoma, tuberculosis, parasitic infestation)

From Henry JB: Clinical Diagnosis and Management by Laboratory Methods, 19th ed. Philadelphia, WB Saunders Co, 1996, p 477.

Table 13–9 □ DIFFERENTIATION OF TRANSUDATIVE
AND EXUDATIVE PLEURAL EFFUSIONS

	Transudate	Exudate
Appearance	Clear, pale yellow	Cloudy, turbid, purulent or bloody
Pleural fluid/serum protein ratio	<0.5	>0.5
Pleural fluid/serum LD ratio	<0.6	>0.6
Pleural fluid cholesterol	<60 mg/dL (<1.55 mmol/L)	>60 mg/dL (>1.55 mmol/L)
Pleural fluid/serum cholesterol ratio	<0.3	>0.3
Pleural fluid/serum bilirubin ratio	<0.6	>0.6

Modified from Kjeldsberg CR, Knight JA: Body Fluids: Laboratory Examination of Amniotic, Cerebrospinal, Seminal, Serous and Synovial Fluids, 3rd ed. © American Society of Clinical Pathologists, Chicago, 1993.
Values in parentheses are SI units.

The classification of casts is made on the basis of composition and origin, as follows.

Hyaline Casts

Hyaline casts are formed by precipitation of protein in the tubular lumen comparable to gel formation, e.g., a sudden change from a fluid to a viscous, semisolid gel. RBC, WBC, and epithelial cells may become trapped in gelatinized casts.

Simple hyaline cast—contains no inclusions and has a refractive index nearly identical to surrounding medium and hence almost invisible unless viewed under subdued light with microscope condenser to its lowest adjustment point.

Hyaline cellular cast—has trapped within, epithelial, red, or white blood cells between which the hyaline stroma may be seen.

Hyaline granular cast—contains granular cellular debris originating from the degeneration of desquamative cellular material from renal tubular epithelial cells.

Hyaline fatty cast—contains highly refractile fat droplets and are usually seen with tubular disease associated with tubular cell deposition of fat and lipid material.

Hyaline casts dissolve in a slightly alkaline medium and hypotonic solution, hence the importance of a fresh specimen, acid pH, and concentrated urine; otherwise these may not be seen in advanced renal disease with inability to concentrate and acidify urine.

Epithelial Casts

Epithelial casts are formed by the conglutination of desquamated necrotic cells from the epithelial lining of the tubule. When first formed, it is a cellular cast; the cells then begin to disintegrate with loss of all margins and dispersion of nuclear material to form a coarsely granular cast and subsequently a finely granular cast. Further disintegration of cellular debris results in a homogeneous mass with a high refractive index called a "waxy cast." Fatty casts characteristic of degenerative tubular disease are a result of fatty degeneration of tubular epithelium in situ with desquamated tubule cells containing droplets of fat, which are often included in hyaline and epithelial casts.

Blood Casts

Blood casts have a characteristic orange-yellow color.

Red blood cell cast—is composed of a solid mass of conglutinated red blood cells tightly packed.

True blood cast—texture is completely homogeneous, and no RBC cell margins can be distinguished (glomerulitis). With local diminution of urinary flow, a red blood cell cast undergoes degeneration to form a *homogeneous true blood cast.* Pathogenesis may relate to glomerulonephritis, embolic glomerulitis, lupus erythematosus, polyarteritis nodosa, and sarcoidosis. Less frequently, they may be observed in toxic nephrosis or renal ischemia syndrome. Rarely, blood casts may appear in urine with gout or chronic pyelonephritis.

Broad Casts or Renal Failure Casts

The appearance of broad casts in any number indicates azotemia or uremia. They are usually epithelial and often waxy but may be of almost any type including hyaline casts.

14

CYTOGENETICS AND MOLECULAR PATHOLOGY

SPECIMEN REQUIREMENTS AND HANDLING
COMMON CYTOGENETIC ABNORMALITIES IN HEMATOLOGIC
  NEOPLASMS

The role of cytogenetics and molecular pathology in clinical medicine is expanding by leaps and bounds. Consequently the availability of these techniques is increasing, and pathologists are expected to be able to appropriately process specimens and report results, either in their own or from reference laboratories. Thus, specimen handling is a crucial part of these determinations, similar to most others, and may be the only procedure many pathologists are asked to perform on call.

■ SPECIMEN REQUIREMENTS AND HANDLING

These are summarized in Table 14–1. Review of your own SOP (standard operating procedures) may be required because these procedures are followed in our laboratory and may differ somewhat from those followed in other laboratories. If specimens have to be sent to a reference laboratory, their recommended procedures (SOPs) must be followed for specimen collection, processing, and transport. It is essential that specimens for cytogenetic analysis be made available to the laboratory as quickly as possible to ensure maximum cell viability.

The list of tests in molecular pathology is, necessarily, partial. The number of abnormalities that can be identified at the molecular level is growing exponentially, and no single laboratory can claim to perform each and every one. Molecular pathology also includes many assays that are approved for research use and should not be used as the sole diagnostic criterion for patient management. This is usually reflected in the report generated by the laboratory and should be made clear to the ordering physician. The rules for patient consent are variable, and our laboratory routinely requires specific signed patient consent forms for such measurements and examinations.

Table 14–1 □ SPECIMEN REQUIREMENTS FOR SELECTED TESTS IN CYTOGENETICS AND MOLECULAR PATHOLOGY

Test	Specimen	Comments
Amniotic fluid karyotype	15–20 mL of amniotic fluid in sterile container	Transport at room temperature
Bone marrow karyotype	1–2 mL of first aspirate in sterile sodium heparinized (green-topped) tube	Transport at room temperature
Peripheral blood karyotype	3–5 mL (adults), 2–3 mL (newborns) of whole blood in sterile sodium heparinized (green-topped) tube	Transport at room temperature
Solid tissue karyotype	Small biopsy specimen placed into sterile medium (Ham's F-10, Dubecco's MEM, RPMI1640)	Do not place in saline solution. Transport on wet ice
Fluorescent in situ hybridization (FISH)	3–5 mL (adults), 2–3 mL (newborns) of whole blood; 1–2 mL of first bone marrow aspirate in sterile sodium heparinized (green-topped) tube	
Alpha-1-antitrypsin deficiency	*Peripheral blood:* 20 mL in EDTA (purple-topped) tubes	Test performed by PCR. Transport at room temperature
Cystic fibrosis	*Peripheral blood:* 20 mL in EDTA (purple-topped) tubes. *Prenatal diagnosis:* cultured amniocytes	Test performed by PCR. Transport at room temperature
Factor V Leiden	*Peripheral blood:* 20 mL in EDTA (purple-topped) tubes	Test performed by PCR. Transport at room temperature

Table 14–1 □ **SPECIMEN REQUIREMENTS FOR SELECTED TESTS IN CYTOGENETICS AND MOLECULAR PATHOLOGY** *Continued*

Test	Specimen	Comments
Fragile X syndrome	*Peripheral blood:* 20 mL in EDTA (purple-topped) tubes *Prenatal diagnosis:* cultured amniocytes	Test performed by PCR and Southern blot Transport at room temperature
Hereditary hemochromatosis	*Peripheral blood:* 20 mL in EDTA (purple-topped) tubes	Test performed by PCR Transport at room temperature
Prothrombin mutation	*Peripheral blood:* 20 mL in EDTA (purple-topped) tubes	Test performed by PCR Transport at room temperature
Sickle cell anemia, hemoglobin C disease	*Peripheral blood:* 20 mL in EDTA (purple-topped) tubes *Prenatal diagnosis:* cultured amniocytes	Test performed by PCR Transport at room temperature
Immunoglobulin gene rearrangement	*Bone marrow:* in sodium heparinized (green-topped) tube *Fresh tissue* *Peripheral blood:* 20–40 mL in sodium heparinized (green-topped) tubes *Formalin-fixed tissue blocks*	Test performed by PCR and Southern blot Transport at room temperature
T-cell receptor gene rearrangement	*Bone marrow:* in sodium heparinized (green-topped) tube *Fresh tissue* *Peripheral blood:* 20–40 mL in sodium heparinized (green-topped) tubes *Formalin-fixed tissue blocks*	Test performed by PCR and Southern blot Transport at room temperature

PCR = polymerase chain reaction

■ COMMON CYTOGENETIC ABNORMALITIES

The common cytogenetic abnormalities are summarized in Tables 14–2 and 14–3.

Table 14–2 □ COMMON CYTOGENETIC ABNORMALITIES IN HEMATOLOGIC DISORDERS

Disease	Cytogenetic Abnormality	Genes Involved
Myelodysplastic syndromes	−5 or del(5q), −7 or del(7q), +8, +9, +19, del(11q), del(12)(p11p13), del(13q), del(20)(q11q13), t(1;3)(p36;q21.2)	
AML (acute myeloblastic leukemia)	+8, −7 or del(7q), −5 or del(5q), t(6;9)(p23;q34)	
AML-M2	t(8;21)(q22;q22)	ETO/AML1
AML-M3	t(15;17)(q22;q11)	PML/RARA
AML-M4Eo	inv(16)(p13q22), t(16;16)(p13;q22)	MYH11/CBFB
AML-M5	t(9;11)(p22;q23)	AF9/MLL
Therapy-related AML	−5 or del(5q), −7 or del(7q), der(1)t(1;7)(p11;p11)	
Biphenotypic (B-ALL/myeloid)	t(4;11)(q21;p23)	AF4/MLL
ALL (acute lymphoblastic leukemia)	Hyperdiploidy (50–60 chromosomes) (good prognosis), hyperdiploid (47–50 chromosomes) (intermediate prognosis), hypodiploid, del(6q), t or del(9p), t or del(12p)	
Precursor B ALL	t(9;22)(q34;q11) t(12;21)(q12;q22) t(4;11)(q21;p23) t(11;19)(q23;p13.3) t(1;19)(q23;p13)	ABL/BCR TEL/AML1 AF4/MLL MLL PBX1/TCF3
B-cell ALL	t(8;14)(q24;q32) t(2;8)(p12;q24) t(8;22)(q24;q1)	MYC/IGH IGK/MYC MYC/IGL

**Table 14–2 □ COMMON CYTOGENETIC ABNORM...
IN HEMATOLOGIC DISORDERS** *Continued*

Disease	Cytogenetic Abnormality	Genes Involved
T-ALL	t(11;14)(p15;q11)	RBTN1/TCRA
	t(11;14)(p13;q11)	RBTN2/TCRA
	t(8;14)(q24;q11)	MYC/TCRA
	inv(14)(q11q32),	TCRA/IGH
	t(14;v)(q11;v), t(7;v)(q34;v),	
	t(7;v)(p15;v)	
CML	t(9;22)(q34;q11)	ABL/BCR
B-CLL	+12	
	t(11;14)(q13;q32)	CCND1/IGH
	t(14;19)(q32;q13)	IGH/BCL3
	t(2;14)(p13;q32)	IGH
T-CLL	inv(14)(q11q32)	TCRA/IGH
Burkitt's	t(8;14)(q24;q32)	MYC/IGH
lymphoma	t(2;8)(p12;q24)	IGK/MYC
	t(8;22)(q24;q1)	MYC/IGL
B-cell follicular lymphoma	t(14;18)(q32;q21)	IGH/BCL2
Diffuse large cell lymphoma		
B-cell large cell	t(3;22)(q27;q11)	BCL6/IGL
lymphoma	t(3;14)(q27;q32)	BCL6/IGH
	t(3q27)	BCL6
Mantle cell lymphoma	t(11;14)(q13;q32)	CCND1/IGH
Lymphoplasmacytoid lymphoma	t(9;14)(p13;q32)	PAX5/IGH
B-cell small lymphocytic lymphoma	t(14;19)(q32;q13)	IGH/BCL3
MALT lymphoma	t(11;18)(q21;q21)	
Anaplastic large cell lymphoma	t(2;5)(p23;q35)	ALK/NPM
Cutaneous T-cell lymphoma	t(10q24)	LYT10
Adult T-cell leukemia or lymphoma	t(14;14)(q11;q32)	TCRA/IGH

CLL = chronic lymphocytic leukemia; CML = chronic myelogenous leukemia; MALT = mucosa-associated lymphoid tissue

SELECTED CYTOGENETIC ABNORMALITIES IN SOLID TUMORS

	Cytogenetic Abnormality	Genes Involved
	t(11;22)(q24;q12)	EWS/FLI1
	t(21;22)(q12;q12)	EWS/ERG
	t(7;22)(p22;q12)	EWS/ETV1
Desmoplastic small round cell tumor	t(11;22)(p13;q12)	EWS/WT1
Alveolar rhabdomyosarcoma	t(2;13)(q35;q14)	PAX3/FKHR
	t(1;13)(p36;q14)	PAX7/FKHR
Synovial sarcoma	t(X;18)(p11;q11)	SYT/SSX1, SYT/SSX2
Clear cell sarcoma	t(12;22)(q13;q12)	EWS/AFT1
Myxoid and round cell liposarcoma	t(12;16)(q13;p11)	TLS/FUS-CHOP
Myxoid chondrosarcoma	t(9;22)(q22;q12)	
Endometrial stromal sarcoma	t(7;17)(p15–21;q12–21)	
Neuroblastoma	Hyperdiploid (good prognosis), del(1p36.2–3) (poor prognosis)	

COMMON CALLS IN
ANATOMIC PATHOLOGY

15

INTRAOPERATIVE CONSULTATION

THE SURGEON'S QUESTION
THE PATHOLOGIST'S RESPONSE
  Clinical History
  Gross Examination
  Frozen Sections
  Cytology
  Special Techniques and Protocols
COMMUNICATING RESULTS

Requests for pathologist's consultation during surgery stem from many different queries, but a common thread that runs through all such consultations is the need for speed and accuracy. The patient, most often, is under anesthesia while the consultation proceeds, hence the emphasis on speed. The pathologist's response may modify the course of surgery or prompt additional procedures and thus the need for accuracy. Many different techniques may be applied for this purpose, most often the examination of frozen sections. The technique of performing frozen sections is learned through practice, but the approach to intraoperative consultations (IOC) in general should be clear before one confronts the surgeon.

■ THE SURGEON'S QUESTION

It is imperative to clearly and comprehensively understand what the surgeon wants. The direct question, "What do you want to know from this IOC?" is often valuable in clarifying this point. Do not be under the impression that the nature of the specimen will make the question obvious; often that is far from the case. A face-to-face conversation with the surgeon in the operating room is ideal; however, in many institutions tissue for IOC is delivered to the pathology department with a requisition form, and the surgeon is available only at the other end of a telephone or intercom. Some of the most common reasons for obtaining an IOC are:

• To establish the diagnosis of an unknown lesion, e.g., a pancreatic mass
• To confirm the nature of excised tissue, e.g., a parathyroid gland

- To confirm adequate (clear) surgical margins in cancer surgery, e.g., basal cell carcinoma
- To evaluate viability of margins, e.g., bowel resection for ischemia
- To ensure that adequate viable tissue is available for a definitive diagnosis, e.g., necrotic tumors
- To submit tissue for special protocols, e.g., lymph node protocol
- To document gross findings in fresh tissue, e.g., distance of colon cancer from colectomy margins

■ THE PATHOLOGIST'S RESPONSE

Many different techniques can be used in responding to an IOC. The most common of these is the frozen section. Many different individuals may be involved in processing and preparing tissue for examination during the IOC. A plan should be formulated early on to allow for a prompt and complete response. Without adequate tissue, it is impossible to make a clinically significant diagnosis. Additional tissue should be requested in such circumstances, and the pathologist should not be pressured by the surgeon into making a diagnosis on inadequate material.

Clinical History

Access to the patient's medical record during an IOC allows the pathologist to get clinical history without having to quiz the surgeon at length. A brief review of the chart to identify major medical and surgical problems and the purpose of the surgery can help the pathologist in formulating a plan for the IOC. Results of prior pathologic examinations from other hospitals may also be contained in the chart and can be valuable in narrowing down a differential diagnosis based on examination of the tissue.

Gross Examination

Although it may not be possible to dictate or write a detailed gross description in the limited time allowed for an IOC, a comprehensive gross examination must be performed. Attributes likely to change after fixation, such as organ weight, dimensions, and distances of tumor from surgical margins, should be recorded. Sutures or other orienting marks should be identified. Significant surgical margins should be inked before the tissue is cut in any way. In some cases, the surgeon may call the pathologist for an IOC simply to hand over the fresh tissue so that it is handled appropriately.

Frozen Sections

Examination of histologic sections of frozen tissue is invaluable in establishing the diagnosis of unknown lesions and in assessing surgical margins. The portion of the tissue to be frozen and its orientation should be determined carefully. Tissue should be covered with freezing medium and frozen rapidly to prevent the formation of ice crystals, which distort the morphologic appearance of cells. This is best accomplished in a isopentane bath precooled in liquid nitrogen. Tissue may be placed directly into liquid nitrogen (care should be taken to avoid splashes), or aerosolized coolants may be used. Placing tissue in the cryostat to freeze is suboptimal, since it is a slow process; it can be speeded up, however, by the use of a metallic heat sink. The aerosolized coolant and heat sink may also be used to cool the surface of the frozen block further if the tissue is fatty, hemorrhagic, or necrotic and does not cut well. Sections should be fixed rapidly in alcohol or formalin to prevent drying of tissue and are then stained with hematoxylin and eosin. Meticulous attention should be paid to labeling specimens and slides appropriately, especially when more than one case is being handled at the same time.

Cytology

Cytologic examination is an excellent adjunct to frozen sections in an IOC and, indeed, is the method of choice in some centers. Several techniques for cytologic preparation are available. These include scrape preparations (smears), crush preparations, and touch imprints. One prepares smears by scraping the tissue with the tip of a scalpel blade and smearing the material so obtained on a glass slide. Crush preparations are suitable for tiny fragments of tissue, and one prepares them by gently crushing the tissue fragment between two glass slides and then pulling the slides apart. Touch imprints are useful in hematopoietic tissues to avoid crushing delicate cells, and one prepares them by gently touching the cut surface of the tissue to a glass slide after blotting off excess blood. Both air-dried and alcohol-fixed cytologic preparations should be prepared; the former are stained with the Romanowsky type of stains such as Diff-Quik, and the latter are stained with hematoxylin and eosin (readily available in the IOC area). Air-dried smears can be prepared, be stained, and be ready for review within a minute or two and greatly help in reducing the turnaround time for an IOC.

Intraoperative fine-needle aspiration (FNA) is popular with some surgeons. The FNA is performed with the patient under anesthesia, and the results of the FNA are used to guide the surgical procedure performed. These samples may be handled by cytopathologists. Air-dried and alcohol-fixed smears are prepared, stained, and interpreted in the usual manner.

Special Techniques and Protocols

Techniques for rapid immunoperoxidase stains based on cytologic preparations or frozen sections have been described and may have utility in selected instances. Since tissue is received fresh for an IOC, it is an excellent opportunity to allocate portions of it for other special studies either according to preexisting protocols (see Chapter 17) or based on the specific needs of the case.

■ COMMUNICATING RESULTS

It has already been emphasized that results need to be communicated promptly to the surgeon, since the patient is often under anesthesia while an IOC is performed. It is equally important to realize that errors in communication at this stage can critically jeopardize the surgeon's decision. Both oral and written communication with the surgeon is vital. A face-to-face conversation is preferable to one through a telephone or intercom. In any event, the diagnosis should be clearly stated as it appears in the written report and then discussed with the surgeon as appropriate. Often the pathologist may have a hypothesis about the nature of the lesion that cannot be substantiated by the results of the IOC alone. Although the pathologist may be right in the end, speculation should be distinguished from fact when he or she is reporting results of an IOC, and any hypotheses should be clearly defined as such. The written report becomes a part of the patient's permanent medical record. Many pathologists also make a separate note in the patient's chart to underscore their role as consultants in such situations. A record of the turnaround time should be kept and, in fact, is a quality monitor used by several inspecting agencies.

AUTOPSY

The postmortem examination is one of the most important aspects of forensic pathology. Its role in hospital deaths in the absence of medicolegal complications has been questioned in recent years, primarily because of more accurate and detailed clinical diagnoses made possible by newer laboratory tests and imaging modalities. However, a well-performed, clinically oriented autopsy that is completed in a timely fashion still retains a valuable place in clinical practice, in addition to its educational benefits.

The purpose of this chapter is not to go over the various methods that have been described for evisceration and dissection of organs. This has to be customized for each individual case, and several excellent texts and monographs are available on this subject. We aim to discuss the overall approach to a case and present a few specific scenarios that require special considerations.

■ PREPARING FOR AN AUTOPSY

Clinical History

Review of the patient's chart is one of the most important parts of an autopsy. It is imperative to know the clinical history including the clinical cause of death as well as significant past medical and surgical history. All surgical procedures should be noted and the anatomic correlates explored during autopsy. In some cases it may be necessary to modify the usual approach to a case based on pertinent clinical information. The physicians caring for the patient should be contacted. Specific questions that should be addressed at that time include the following:

- What were the clinical problems?
- What was the clinical cause of death?
- What specific clinical questions should the autopsy address? This may include both anatomic and clinical pathologic issues, such as blood and tissue cultures and serologic and chemical studies.
- Would any of the physicians or other persons involved with the patient's care like to be present at autopsy? Within reasonable limits, the pathologist should attempt to accommodate such requests. Specifically in the case of postsurgery autopsies, it is particularly useful to have a member of the surgical team present during autopsy to help with difficult dissections. Calls to physicians and other health care providers should be documented for reference.

Scheduling the Autopsy

Autopsies are usually performed during regular working hours on weekdays or during the day on weekends. It may be necessary to perform at least the evisceration in the evening or at night to accommodate the wishes of the family for an early release of the body to the funeral home or for other reasons. Haste, however, should not result in oversights, and it is important to follow standard protocols at all times.

Autopsy Permit

Verification of a valid autopsy permit is absolutely essential before any procedures are carried out. In many institutions, the permit is obtained by persons other than the pathologist performing the autopsy. It is imperative to verify that an autopsy permit signed by the next of kin or other legal representative is available, and this should be reviewed carefully by the pathologist before the procedure is started. In addition to the person authorizing the autopsy, the permit usually contains the name of the person (physician or other) who sought the permit. This can sometimes help in contacting the physician most interested in the autopsy findings, particularly in the case of patients with complicated medical courses who have been under the care of many different physicians.

Restricted Autopsies

Always check the permit for restrictions to the autopsy. Although the goal of a good autopsy is to examine every organ system and arrive at specific conclusions, boundaries set by the family in the form of restrictions should never be breached for academic purposes. The most frequent restriction is "no CNS" and is easily followed. More stringent restrictions such as "chest only" or "examination through surgical incision only" may lead to a severely restricted autopsy, but usually in such instances the chief clinical questions can be answered. Occasionally one may be faced with a seemingly absurd restriction, such as "no CNS" in a patient dying of CNS disease. In such cases, this issue should be discussed with the physician to determine if there are other significant findings that may be diagnosed from the rest of the case, and perhaps the family should be approached to discuss the reasons for the restriction.

In most cases, especially in academic centers, organs are preserved for subsequent dissection and presentation at conferences. If the family desires all tissues to be replaced in the body, only those pieces of tissue necessary for histologic sampling should be saved.

■ PLANNING THE AUTOPSY

No single protocol can serve every case. Each patient is an individual, and therefore each autopsy has to be individualized to address the problems presented in that case. A protocol should be constructed with the help of the attending pathologist and may be modified as needed during the procedure itself. Consultation with specialist pathologists such as neuropathologists, pediatric pathologists, and pulmonary pathologists may be necessary to plan the procedure to ensure that unexpected or subtle findings are not overlooked. Notes should be made during the procedure to document findings (either an assistant can write down findings or a dictation system can be used) rather than trusting memory.

Special Studies

Special studies may be required in specific cases. There is no complete list of such studies, but the following are some things to be kept in mind:

- *Microbiologic studies*—bacterial, viral, fungal, mycobacterial cultures; special cultures for fastidious or unusual organisms.
- *Chemical analysis and toxicology*—samples include fluids (blood, urine, CSF, vitreous humor, effusion fluids) and tissues (liver, kidney, brain).
- *Serologic or other immunologic tests.*
- *Cytogenetics*—tissue samples depend on the case but should be harvested early so that viable cells can be obtained.

- *Molecular studies*—fresh tissue can be flash frozen and preserved for a variety of molecular tests; many tests can also be carried out on formalin-fixed tissues.
- *Special stains, immunofluorescence, and immunohistochemistry*—tissues may need to be frozen or preserved in special solutions.

Photography

Photographs of autopsy findings in situ are the only permanent visual records of the case and are invaluable in supplementing the written autopsy report in case presentations. All unusual and potentially significant findings should be photographed if possible. Photographs of dissected organs showing the main findings are also recommended and can be obtained after the evisceration is completed.

Histologic Sections

There is no correct number of histologic sections, and each case is necessarily unique. The autopsy is a wonderful tool to learn normal histology in addition to pathologic histology, and hence it is recommended that all major organs be sampled for histologic characteristics. Obviously, pathologic processes must be documented first, before grossly normal tissues are submitted for histologic analysis. Small pieces of multiple organs with no gross abnormality can be submitted in a single cassette to be economical. The following is a general list of tissues that may be submitted for histologic analysis when organs are otherwise grossly normal:

- *Cardiovascular system*—right and left ventricular wall, interventricular septum, coronary arteries, aorta
- *Lungs*—sections from each lobe including peripheral lung with pleura and central lung with large airways
- *Hepatobiliary system*—right and left lobe of liver, gallbladder
- *Pancreas*—head and body
- *Spleen*
- *Gastrointestinal tract*—sections from each part or junctional sections (gastroesophageal junction, pylorus and duodenum, ileocecal valve)
- *Kidneys*—right and left, showing cortex, medulla, and collecting system
- *Urinary bladder*
- *Endocrine system*—adrenals, thyroid, pituitary
- *Male reproductive system*—prostate, testis
- *Female reproductive system*—uterus, cervix, ovaries
- *Lymph nodes*—mediastinal, retroperitoneal
- *Bone marrow*

- *Central nervous system*—multiple sections of cerebral cortex, basal ganglia, hippocampus, midbrain, pons, medulla, cervical spinal cord

Tissue samples from skin, peripheral nerve, and skeletal muscle should be collected in each case though they need not be routinely processed for histologic analysis. Judicious use of histologic sections is essential, and most cases should not have more than 20 blocks (excluding CNS). Since this is the same number of blocks as may be expected from a complicated surgical case, there is no reason for the histology lab to delay processing the autopsy (as may happen if autopsy cases routinely yield 30 or more blocks).

■ AUTOPSY REPORTS

A provisional anatomic diagnosis must be rendered upon completion of the autopsy based on the clinical and gross pathologic findings. This should be discussed with the attending pathologist and completed immediately after the autopsy is finished. This is usually required before the body can be released to the funeral home.

The preliminary autopsy report, which details the clinical and gross autopsy findings, should be completed within 48 hours. This is the first written communication to the patient's physicians and should address all major clinical concerns. Although this is essentially based on gross findings, occasionally a few selected tissue sections may aid greatly in arriving at a more definitive diagnosis. In such cases, some blocks should be rush processed through histologic analysis if the usual procedure in the histology lab is not to process autopsy cases the day they are submitted.

The final autopsy report is completed after review of the histologic sections and completion of special studies. The completed report should include a summary of the clinical course of the patient, gross autopsy findings (external and internal examination), microscopic descriptions of histologic sections, results of special studies, and the final autopsy diagnosis. Although most hospitals allow as much as 30 days or more for completing final autopsy reports, in uncomplicated cases this requirement is easily accomplished in 4 or 5 days. Timely autopsy reports have a much greater effect on the treating physicians and greatly enhance the value of the autopsy.

Final autopsy reports are routinely sent to physicians involved in the patient's care and to medical records. They may be requested by the family of the deceased, and this must be kept in mind when one is writing the report. Some institutions incorporate a brief summary written in lay terms to allow the family members to better understand the content of the report.

SPECIAL PROTOCOLS

LYMPH NODE PROTOCOL
KIDNEY BIOPSY
SKELETAL MUSCLE BIOPSY
PERIPHERAL NERVE BIOPSY
IMMUNOFLUORESCENCE STUDIES
TISSUE FOR DRUG-RESISTANCE STUDIES

Several special protocols in anatomic pathology allow expeditious and efficient handling of tissue specimens ensuring that all necessary tests can be performed in the most optimal fashion. This may include special tissue handling, use of special fixatives, and partitioning of tissue for multiple different anticipated studies, which may involve several different laboratories.

■ LYMPH NODE PROTOCOL

A systematic approach to hematologic tissues obtained for the purpose of evaluating hematopoietic malignancies and other disorders involves many different diagnostic tools, and therefore a standardized protocol is valuable. This protocol is used for lymph node biopsies and for other hematopoietic tissues such as spleen and tonsils. Surgeons should be encouraged to inform the pathology department in advance when a lymph node protocol would be required to allow necessary preparations to be made.

The most crucial aspect of lymphoma diagnosis is the availability of well-fixed and well-stained histologic sections. The use of special fixatives such as B5 (mercury based) or Z-Fix (zinc based) allow better visualization of nuclear detail. Fixatives are discussed further in Appendix B. Ancillary studies that may be required include immunohistochemistry (which is dependent on adequate fixation of fresh tissue), flow cytometry for surface markers, cytogenetics, electron microscopy, molecular studies, microbiologic cultures, and others. Although each of these may not be involved in every case, it is often impossible to predict which ones will be needed. Thus it is prudent to save specimens for all these possible needs, if sufficient tissue is available.

The specimen should be collected fresh and in a sterile environment from the surgeon. To prevent drying, one may place the tissue on a sterile gauze pad soaked with sterile saline. However, the specimen should not be immersed in saline. The tissue is then handled as follows:

- *Microbiologic studies (if indicated)*. Tissue for microbiology should be collected under strict sterile conditions and is best done by the surgeon before the specimen is given to the pathologist. If the pathologist is separating tissue for microbiology, sterile instruments should be used, and tissue for microbiology should be separated before any of the other procedures.
- *Touch imprints*. Five to 10 touch imprints should be prepared from multiple different cut faces of the tissue. The tissue should be gently touched to the slide (after excess blood is blotted off) to prevent a crush artifact. These slides are air dried and stained with Wright-Giemsa stain.
- *Routine histology*
  - Formalin fixed—one or two thin slices.
  - B5 fixed—one or two thin slices; fix for 2 hours (never more than 4 hours) and then transfer to formalin.
  - These specimens are used for routine immunohistochemistry.
- *Electron microscopy (EM)*. Glutaraldehyde or other fixative—several 1 mm^3 pieces for optimal fixation.
- *Flow cytometry*. Fresh tissue is placed into tissue culture medium (such as RPMI1640) and stored in the refrigerator if not processed immediately.
- *Cytogenetics*. Fresh tissue is placed into tissue culture medium (such as RPMI1640, Ham's F-10) and stored in the refrigerator if not processed immediately.
- *Other studies*.
  - Tissue is flash frozen in liquid nitrogen and stored at $-70°C$ for special molecular tests, immunofluorescence, and immunohistochemistry.

If adequate tissue is not available, routine histologic analysis and flow cytometry are most important for diagnosing hematopoietic malignancies.

■ KIDNEY BIOPSY

Renal biopsy specimens are routinely processed for light microscopy (including special stains), immunofluorescence, and electron microscopy. Glomerular disease cannot be demonstrated if renal cortex is not sampled; therefore the adequacy of tissue should be assessed before the tissue is processed. If multiple cores are available, one core is frozen for immunofluorescence studies, one or more cores are placed in formalin, and 1-mm pieces from the ends of one or more cores are placed in EM fixative. If only a single core is available, as is often the case, a dissecting microscope should be used to ascertain the presence of cortical and medullary tissue in the core. A 1-mm piece from the cortical end (containing glomeruli) is submitted for EM, and the remaining tissue is split lengthwise, one portion used for immunofluorescence and one portion fixed in formalin.

The procedure above requires handling of fresh tissue. If this is not possible, two cores may be obtained, one placed in Zamboni's solution (for light microscopy and EM) and one placed in Michel's solution (for immunofluorescence). These fixatives are stable at room temperature and may be used to transport specimens to a renal pathologist. Renal biopsy specimens from transplanted kidneys for the purpose of diagnosing rejection need not be submitted for EM and immunofluorescence in most cases.

■ SKELETAL MUSCLE BIOPSY

Skeletal muscle biopsy specimens should be placed in a muscle clamp to prevent contraction. The specimen should be handled promptly to avoid degradation of muscle enzymes, which form a major part in the diagnosis of muscle disease. A portion of the muscle is snap frozen and used for enzyme histochemical stains and chemical analysis. This is a crucial step, and slow freezing must be avoided to ensure satisfactory stains. An isopentane bath precooled in liquid nitrogen may be used for this purpose. Additionally, small pieces of muscle (1 mm^3 each) are submitted for EM, and some formalin-fixed tissue (in both longitudinal and cross-sectional orientation) is submitted for routine histologic analysis.

■ PERIPHERAL NERVE BIOPSY

The sural nerve is most commonly biopsied for this purpose. The surgeon may request an intraoperative consultation to confirm the presence of peripheral nerve tissue; for this purpose a crush smear or frozen section performed on a 1- to 2-mm fragment from the tip of the specimen is adequate. Tissue for immunofluorescence studies (if needed) should be separated first and frozen or submitted in Michel's fixative. The nerve should be pinned to a corkboard with minimal manipulation and fixed before further handling, since the fresh tissue is easily crushed and damaged. Fixation in glutaraldehyde is preferred, since this also prepares the tissue for EM. After fixation for at least 1 hour, multiple cross sections are made from the central portion of the nerve and submitted for EM. Additionally, pieces are submitted in formalin for histologic analysis in both longitudinal and cross-sectional orientation. Tissue for EM is most important in nerve biopsy interpretation and should be procured first.

■ IMMUNOFLUORESCENCE STUDIES

Skin and other tissue specimens for immunofluorescence should be received fresh, on saline-moistened gauze to prevent drying. Tissue for immunofluorescence is frozen and stored at $-70°C$ or placed into Michel's solution and stored at room temperature. A portion of the tissue may be submitted in formalin for routine histologic analysis for morphologic evaluation. Skin punch biopsy specimens are generally bisected (with care being taken to include lesional tissue in both halves); one half is submitted for immunofluorescence and the other for routine histologic analysis.

■ TISSUE FOR DRUG-RESISTANCE STUDIES

Studies for resistance to chemotherapeutic drugs are available for solid tumors and are used most often in gynecologic malignancies. Tissue must be obtained under sterile conditions and is submitted in culture medium provided by the laboratory performing the test. It is essential to have viable tissue for the study, and a frozen-section examination may be indicated to confirm viability. The ability to render a histologic diagnosis must not be compromised in any way when the tissue is sent for such studies, and therefore the attending pathologist should be consulted before tissue is submitted for such studies.

APPENDIX A

□ □ □

REFERENCE INTERVALS
(NORMAL VALUES)
AND SI UNITS

A–1 □ WHOLE BLOOD, SERUM, AND PLASMA CHEMISTRY

Typical Reference Intervals

Component	System	Conventional Units	Factor*	Recommended SI Units†
Acetoacetic acid				
qualitative	Serum	Negative	—	Negative
quantitative	Serum	0.2–1.0 mg/dL	97.95	20–100 μmol/L
Acetone				
qualitative	Serum	Negative	—	Negative
quantitative	Serum	0.3–2.0 mg/dL	172.95	20–340 μmol/L
Albumin				
qualitative	Serum	3.2–4.5 g/dL (salt fractionation)	10	32–45 g/L
		3.2–5.6 g/dL (electrophoresis)		32–56 g/L
		3.8–5.0 g/dL (dye binding)		38–50 g/L
Alcohol, ethyl	Serum or whole blood	Negative—but presented as mg/dL	0.2171	Negative—but presented as mmol/L
Aldolase	Serum			
	adults	3–8 Sibley-Lehinger U/dL at 37°C	7.4	22–59 mU/L at 37°C
	children	Approximately 2 times adult levels		Approximately 2 times adult levels
	newborn	Approximately 4 times adult levels		Approximately 4 times adult levels
α-Amino acid nitrogen	Serum	3.6–7.0 mg/dL	0.7139	2.6–5.0 mmol/L
δ-Aminolevulinic acid	Serum	0.01–0.03 mg/dL	76.26	0.8–2.3 μmol/L

Table continued on following page

See footnotes on p. 284.

A–1 □ WHOLE BLOOD, SERUM, AND PLASMA CHEMISTRY *Continued*

Component	System	Typical Reference Intervals		
		Conventional Units	*Factor**	*Recommended SI Units†*
Ammonia	Plasma	20–120 μg/dL (diffusion)	0.5872	12–70 μmol/L
		40–80 μg/dL (enzymatic method)		23–47 μmol/L
		12–48 μg/dL (resin method)		7–28 μmol/L
Amylase	Serum	16–120 Somogyi units/dL	1.85	30–220 U/L
Argininosuccinate lyase	Serum	0–4 U/dL	10	0–40 U/L
Arsenic‡	Whole blood	<7 μg/dL	0.05055	<0.4 μmol/L
Ascorbic acid (vitamin C)	Plasma	0.6–1.6 mg/dL	56.78	34–91 μmol/L
	Whole blood	0.7–2.0 mg/dL		40–114 μmol/L
Barbiturates	Serum, plasma, or whole blood	Negative	—	Negative
Base excess	Whole blood			
male		−3.3 to +1.2 mEq/L	1	−3.3 to +1.2 mmol/L
female		−2.4 to +2.3 mEq/L		−2.4 to +2.3 mmol/L
Base, total	Serum	145–160 mEq/L	1	145–160 mmol/L
Bicarbonate	Plasma	21–28 mmol/L	1	21–28 mmol/L
Bile acids	Serum	0.3–3.0 mg/dL	10	3.0–30.0 mg/L
Bilirubin	Serum		17.10	
direct (conjugated)		<0.3 mg/dL		<5 μmol/L
indirect (unconjugated)		0.1–1.0 mg/dL		2–17 μmol/L
total		0.1–1.2 mg/dL		2–21 μmol/L
newborns, total		1.0–12.0 mg/dL		17–205 μmol/L

Blood gases (see Chap. 12)

pH	Whole blood	7.38–7.44 (arterial)	1	7.38–7.44
		7.36–7.41 (venous)		7.36–7.41
P_{CO_2}	Whole blood	35–40 mm Hg (arterial)	0.1333	4.7–5.3 kPa
		40–45 mm Hg (venous)		5.3–6.0 kPa
P_{O_2}	Whole blood	95–100 mm Hg (arterial)	0.1333	12.7–13.3 kPa
Bromide	Serum	<5 mg/dL	0.125	<0.63 mmol/L
Calcium				
ionized	Serum	4.0–4.8 mg/dL	0.2500	1.00–1.20 mmol/L
		2.0–2.4 mEq/L	0.5000	
		30–58% of total	0.01	0.30–1.58 of total
total	Serum	9.2–11.0 mg/dL	0.2500	2.30–2.74 mmol/L
		4.6–5.5 mEq/L	0.5000	
Carbon dioxide (CO_2 content)	Whole blood (arterial)	19–24 mmol/L	1	19–24 mmol/L
	Plasma or serum (arterial)	21–28 mmol/L		21–28 mmol/L
Carbon dioxide	Whole blood (venous)	22–26 mmol/L	1	22–26 mmol/L
	Plasma or serum (venous)	24–30 mmol/L		24–30 mmol/L
CO_2 combining power	Plasma or serum (venous)	24–30 mmol/L	1	24–30 mmol/L
CO_2 partial pressure (P_{CO_2})	Whole blood (arterial)	35–40 mm Hg	0.1333	4.7–5.3 kPa
	Whole blood (venous)	40–45 mm Hg		5.3–6.0 kPa

Table continued on following page

A–1 □ WHOLE BLOOD, SERUM, AND PLASMA CHEMISTRY *Continued*

		Typical Reference Intervals		
Component	System	Conventional Units	Factor*	Recommended SI Units†
Carbonic acid (H_2CO_3)	Whole blood (arterial)	1.05–1.45 mmol/L	1	1.05–1.45 mmol/L
	Whole blood (venous)	1.15–1.50 mmol/L		1.15–1.50 mmol/L
	Plasma (venous)	1.02–1.38 mmol/L		1.02–1.38 mmol/L
Carboxyhemoglobin (carbon monoxide hemoglobin)	Whole blood	<1.5% saturation of hemoglobin	0.01	Fraction hemoglobin saturated: <0.015
	suburban nonsmokers			
	smokers	1.5–5.0% saturation		0.015–0.050
	heavy smokers	5.0–9.0% saturation		0.050–0.090
Carotene, beta	Serum	40–200 µg/dL	0.01863	0.7–3.7 µmol/L
Ceruloplasmin	Serum	23–50 mg/dL	10	230–500 mg/L
Chloride	Serum	95–103 mEq/L	1	95–103 mmol/L
Cholesterol total (see Chap. 12)	Serum	150–250 mg/dL (varies with diet, sex, and age)	0.02586	3.88–6.47 mmol/L
esters	Serum	65–75% of total cholesterol	0.01	Fraction of total cholesterol: 0.65–0.75
Cholinesterase (pseudocholinesterase)	Erythrocytes	0.65–1.3 pH units	1	0.65–1.3 units§
	Plasma	0.5–1.3 pH units	1	0.5–1.3 units
		8–18 U/L at 37°C		8–18 U/L at 37°C
Citrate	Serum or plasma	1.7–3.0 mg/dL	52.05	88–156 µmol/L

		Conventional	Factor	SI
Copper	Serum, plasma			
	male	70–140 µg/dL	0.1574	11–22 µmol/L
	female	80–155 µg/dL		13–24 µmol/L
Cortisol	Plasma			
	8 A.M.–10 A.M.	5–23 µg/dL	27.59	138–635 nmol/L
	4 P.M.–6 P.M.	3–13 µg/dL		83–359 nmol/L
Creatine	Serum or plasma			
	male	0.1–0.4 mg/dL	76.25	8–31 µmol/L
	female	0.2–0.7 mg/dL		15–53 µmol/L
Creatine kinase (CK)	Serum			
	male	55–170 U/L at 37°C	1	55–170 U/L at 37°C
	female	30–135 U/L at 37°C	1	30–135 U/L at 37°C
Creatinine	Serum or plasma	0.6–1.2 mg/dL (adult)	88.40	53–106 µmol/L
		0.3–0.6 mg/dL (children <2 y)		27–53 µmol/L
Creatinine clearance (endogenous)	Serum or plasma and urine			
	male	107–139 mL/min	0.01667	1.78–2.32 mL/s
	female	87–107 mL/min		1.45–1.78 mL/s
Cryoglobulins	Serum	Negative	—	Negative
Electrophoresis, protein albumin	Serum	52–65% of total protein	0.01	Fraction of total protein: 0.52–0.65
alpha-1		2.5–5.0% of total protein	0.01	0.025–0.05
alpha-2		7.0–13.0% of total protein	0.01	0.07–0.13
beta		8.0–14.0% of total protein	0.01	0.08–0.14
gamma		12.0–22.0% of total protein	0.01	0.12–0.22

Table continued on following page

A–1 □ WHOLE BLOOD, SERUM, AND PLASMA CHEMISTRY *Continued*

Component	System	Conventional Units	Factor*	Recommended SI Units†
Electrophoresis, protein *Continued*	Serum	Concentration		
albumin		3.2–5.6 g/dL	10	32–56 g/L
alpha-1		0.1–0.4 g/dL		1–4 g/L
alpha-2		0.4–1.2 g/dL		4–12 g/L
beta		0.5–1.1 g/dL		5–11 g/L
gamma		0.5–1.6 g/dL		5–16 g/L
Fats, neutral (see Triglycerides)				
Fatty acids				
total (free and esterified)	Serum	9–15 mmol/L	1	9–15 mmol/L
free (nonesterified)	Plasma	300–480 µEq/L	1	300–480 µmol/L
Ferritin	Serum			
male		15–200 ng/mL	1	15–200 µg/L
female		12–150 ng/mL	1	15–150 µg/L
Fibrinogen	Plasma	200–400 mg/dL	0.01	2.00–4.00 g/L
Fluoride	Whole blood	<0.05 mg/dL	0.5263	<0.027 mmol/L
Folate	Serum	5–25 ng/mL (bioassay)	2.266	11–57 nmol/L
		>2.3 ng/mL (radioassay)		>5 nmol/L
	Erythrocytes	166–640 ng/mL (bioassay)		376–1450 nmol/L
		>140 ng/mL (radioassay)		>317 nmol/L

	Specimen	Conventional	Factor	SI
Galactose	Whole blood adults	None		None
	children	<20 mg/dL	0.05551	<1.11 mmol/L
Gamma globulin	Serum	0.5–1.6 g/dL	10	5–16 g/L
Globulins, total	Serum	2.3–3.5 g/dL	10	23–35 g/L
Glucose, fasting	Serum or plasma	70–110 mg/dL	0.0551	3.9–6.1 mmol/L
	Whole blood	60–100 mg/dL		3.3–5.6 mmol/L
Glucose tolerance	Serum or plasma			
oral	fasting	70–110 mg/dL	0.05551	3.9–6.1 mmol/L
	30 min	30–60 mg/dL above fasting		1.7–3.3 mmol/L above fasting
	60 min	20–50 mg/dL above fasting		1.1–2.8 mmol/L above fasting
	120 min	5–15 mg/dL above fasting		0.3–0.8 mmol/L above fasting
	180 min	Fasting level or below		Fasting level or below
intravenous	Serum or plasma			
	fasting	70–110 mg/dL		3.9–6.1 mmol/L
	5 min	Maximum of 250 mg/dL		Maximum of 13.9 mmol/L
	60 min	Significant decrease		Significant decrease
	120 min	Below 120 mg/dL		Below 6.7 mmol/L
	180 min	Fasting level		Fasting level
Glucose-6-phosphate	Erythrocytes	250–5000 units/10^6 cells	1	250–5000 μunits/cell
dehydrogenase (G6PD)		1200–2000 mIU/mL packed erythrocytes	1	1200–2000 U/L packed erythrocytes
γ-Glutamyltransferase	Serum	5–40 IU/L	1	5–40 U/L at 37°C
Glutathione	Whole blood	24–37 mg/dL	0.03254	0.78–1.20 mmol/L

Table continued on following page

A–1 □ WHOLE BLOOD, SERUM, AND PLASMA CHEMISTRY *Continued*

Component	System	Conventional Units	Factor[a]	Recommended SI Units[†]
				Typical Reference Intervals
Growth hormone	Serum	<10 ng/mL	1	<10 µg/L
Guanase	Serum	<3 nmol/mL/min	1	<3 U/L at 37°C
Haptoglobin	Serum	60–270 mg/dL	0.01	0.6–2.7 g/L
Hemoglobin	Serum or plasma			
qualitative		Negative	—	Negative
quantitative		0.5–5.0 mg/dL	10	5–50 mg/L
	Whole blood			
female		12.0–16.0 g/dL	10	120–160 g/L
male		13.5–18.0 g/dL	10	135–180 g/L
α-Hydroxybutyrate dehydrogenase	Serum	140–350 U/mL	1	140–350 kU/L
17-Hydroxycorticosteroids	Plasma			
male		7–19 µg/dL	25.59‖	193–524 nmol/L
female		9–21 µg/dL		248–579 nmol/L
	after 24 USP units of ACTH I.M.			
	Serum	35–55 µg/dL		966–1517 nmol/L
Immunoglobulins	Serum			
IgG		800–1801 mg/dL	0.01	8.0–18.0 g/L
IgA		113–563 mg/dL		1.1–5.6 g/L
IgM		54–222 mg/dL		0.5–2.2 g/L
IgD		0.5–3.0 mg/dL	10	5.0–30.0 mg/L
IgE		0.01–0.04 mg/dL		0.1–0.4 mg/L

Analyte	Specimen	Reference range (conventional)	Factor	Reference range (SI)
Insulin	Plasma bioassay radioimmunoassay	11–240 µIU/mL 4–24 µIU/mL	7.175††	79–1722 pmol/L 29–172 pmol/L
Insulin tolerance (0.1 unit/kg)	Serum fasting 30 min 90 min	Glucose of 70–110 mg/dL Fall to 50% of fasting level Fasting level	0.05551 0.01	Glucose of 3.9–6.1 mmol/L Fall to 0.5 of fasting level Fasting level
Iron, total	Serum	60–150 µg/dL	0.1791	10.7–26.9 µmol/L
Iron-binding capacity	Serum	250–400 µg/dL	0.1791	44.8–71.6 µmol/L
Iron saturation	Serum	20–55%	0.01	Fraction of total iron-binding capacity: 0.20–0.55
Isocitric dehydrogenase	Serum	50–240 units/mL at 25°C (Wolfson-Williams Ashman units)	0.0166	0.83–4.18 U/L at 25°C
Ketone bodies	Serum	Negative	—	Negative
17-Ketosteroids	Plasma	25–125 µg/dL	34.67¶	866–4334 nmol/L
Lactic acid (as lactate)	Whole blood venous arterial	5–20 mg/dL 3–7 mg/dL	0.1110	0.6–2.2 mmol/L 0.3–0.8 mmol/L
Lactate dehydrogenase (LD)	Serum	(lactate → pyruvate) 80–120 units at 30°C (pyruvate → lactate) 185–640 units at 30°C (lactate → pyruvate) 100–190 U/L at 37°C	0.48 0.48 1	38–62 U/L at 30°C 90–310 U/L at 30°C 100–190 U/L at 37°C

Table continued on following page

A–1 □ WHOLE BLOOD, SERUM, AND PLASMA CHEMISTRY *Continued*

Component	System	Typical Reference Intervals		
		Conventional Units	*Factor**	*Recommended SI Units*†
Lactate dehydrogenase isoenzymes	Serum			Fraction of total LD
LD₁ (anode)		17–27%	0.01	0.17–0.27
LD₂		27–37%		0.27–0.37
LD₃		18–25%		0.18–0.25
LD₄		3–8%		0.03–0.08
LD₅ (cathode)		0–5%		0.00–0.05
Lactate dehydrogenase (heat stable)	Serum	30–60% of total	0.01	Fraction of total LD: 0.30–0.60
Lactose tolerance	Serum	Serum glucose changes similar to glucose tolerance test	—	Serum glucose changes similar to glucose tolerance test
Lead	Whole blood	<50 μg/dL	0.04826	<2.41 μmol/L
Leucine aminopeptidase (LAP)	Serum male	80–200 U/mL (Goldbarg-Rutenberg)	0.24	19.2–48.0 U/L
	female	75–185 U/mL (Goldbarg-Rutenberg)		18.0–44.4 U/L
Lipase	Serum	0–1.5 U/mL (Cherry-Crandall)	278	0–417 U/L
		14–280 mIU/mL	1	14–280 U/L

Analyte	Specimen	Conventional value	Factor	SI value
Lipids, total	Serum	400–800 mg/dL	0.01	4.00–8.00 g/L
cholesterol (see Chap. 12)		150–250 mg/dL	0.02586	3.88–6.47 mmol/L
triglycerides (see Chap.12)		10–90 mg/dL	0.01129**	0.11–2.15 mmol/L
phospholipids		150–380 mg/dL	0.01	1.50–3.80 g/L
fatty acids (free)		9.0–15.0 mmol/L	1	9.0–15.0 mmol/L
phospholipid phosphorus		8.0–11.0 mg/dL	0.3229	2.58–3.55 mmol/L
Lithium	Serum	Negative	—	Negative
therapeutic interval		0.5–1.4 mEq/L	1	0.5–1.4 mmol/L
Long-acting thyroid-stimulating hormone (LATS)	Serum	None detected	—	None detected
Luteinizing hormone (LH)	Serum		1	
male		6–30 mIU/mL		6–30 IU/L
female		Midcycle peak: 3 times baseline value		Midcycle peak: 3 times baseline value
		Premenopausal <30 mIU/mL		Premenopausal <30 IU/L
		Postmenopausal >35 mIU/mL		Postmenopausal >35 IU/L
Macroglobulins, total	Serum	70–430 mg/dL	0.01	0.7–4.3 g/L
Magnesium	Serum	1.3–2.1 mEq/L	0.5000	0.65–1.05 mmol/L
		1.8–3.0 mg/dL	0.4114	0.74–1.23 mmol/L
Methemoglobin	Whole blood	<0.24 g/dL	10	<2.4 g/L
		<1% of total hemoglobin	0.01	Fraction of total hemoglobin <0.01

Table continued on following page

A–1 □ WHOLE BLOOD, SERUM, AND PLASMA CHEMISTRY Continued

Component	System	Conventional Units	Factor*	Recommended SI Units†
			Typical Reference Intervals	
Mucoprotein	Serum	80–200 mg/dL	0.01	0.8–2.0 g/L
Muramidase	Serum	4–13 mg/L		4–13 mg/L
Myoglobin	Serum	<90 μg/L		<90 μg/L
Nonprotein nitrogen (NPN)	Serum or plasma	20–35 mg/dL	0.7139	14.3–25.0 mmol/L
	Whole blood	25–50 mg/dL		17.8–35.7 mmol/L
5'-Nucleotidase	Serum	0–1.6 units at 37°C	1	0–1.6 units at 37°C
Ornithine carbamyl-transferase	Serum	8–20 mIU/mL at 37°C	1	8–20 U/L at 37°C
Osmolality	Serum	280–295 mOsm/kg	1	280–295 mmol/kg
Oxygen pressure (Po₂)	Whole blood (arterial)	95–100 mm Hg	0.1333	12.7–13.3 kPa
content	Whole blood (arterial)	15–23 volume %	0.01	Volume fraction: 0.15–0.23
saturation	Whole blood (arterial)	94–100%		Fraction saturated: 0.94–1.00
pH	Whole blood (arterial)	7.38–7.44	1	7.38–7.44
	Whole blood (venous)	7.36–7.41		7.36–7.41
	Serum or plasma (venous)	7.35–7.45		7.35–7.45

Phenylalanine	Serum			
	adults	<3.0 mg/dL	60.54	<182 μmol/L
	newborns (term)	1.2–3.5 mg/dL		73–212 μmol/L
Phosphatase				
acid phosphatase	Serum	0.13–0.63 U/L at 37°C	16.67	2.2–10.5 U/L at 37°C
		(p-nitrophenyl phosphate)		
alkaline phosphatase	Serum	20–130 IU/L at 37°C	1	20–130 U/L at 37°C
		(p-nitrophenyl phosphate		
		in AMP buffer)		
Phospholipid phosphorus				
(see Lipids, total)				
Phospholipids				
(see Lipids, total)				
Phosphorus, inorganic	Serum			
	adults	2.3–4.7 mg/dL	0.3229	0.74–1.52 mmol/L
	children	4.0–7.0 mg/dL		1.29–2.26 mmol/L
Potassium	Plasma	3.8–5.0 mEq/L		3.8–5.0 mmol/L
Prolactin	Serum female	1–25 ng/mL	1	1–25 μg/L
	male	1–20 ng/mL	1	1–20 μg/L
Proteins	Serum			
total		6.0–7.8 g/dL	10	60–78 g/L
albumin		3.2–4.5 g/dL		32–45 g/L
globulin		2.3–3.5 g/dL		23–35 g/L
Protein fractionation		See Electrophoresis		See Electrophoresis
Protoporphyrin	Erythrocytes	15–50 mg/dL	0.01777	0.27–0.89 μmol/L
Pyruvate	Whole blood	0.3–0.9 mg/dL	113.6	34–102 μmol/L

Table continued on following page

A–1 □ WHOLE BLOOD, SERUM, AND PLASMA CHEMISTRY *Continued*

Component	System	Typical Reference Intervals		
		Conventional Units	*Factor**	*Recommended SI Units†*
Salicylates	Serum			
therapeutic interval		15–30 mg/dL	0.07240	1.08–2.17 mmol/L
Sodium	Plasma	136–142 mEq/L	1	136–142 mmol/L
Sulfate, inorganic	Serum	0.2–1.3 mEq/L	0.5	0.10–0.65 mmol/L
		0.9–6.0 mg/dL as $SO_4^=$	0.1042	0.09–0.63 mmol/L as $SO_4^=$
Sulfhemoglobin	Whole blood	Negative	—	Negative
Sulfonamides	Serum or whole blood	Negative	—	Negative
Testosterone	Serum or plasma			
	male	300–1200 ng/dL	0.03467	10.4–41.6 nmol/L
	female	30–95 ng/dL		1.0–3.3 nmol/L
Thiocyanate	Serum	Negative	—	Negative
Thyroid hormone tests	Serum			
thyroxine, total (T_4)		5.5–12.5 µg/dL	12.87	71–161 nmol/L
thyroxine, free (FT_4)		0.9–2.3 ng/dL	12.87	12–30 pmol/L
T_3 resin uptake		25–38 relative % uptake	0.01	Relative uptake fraction: 0.25–0.38
thyroxine-binding globulin (TBG)	Serum	10–26 µg/dL	10	100–260 µg/L
thyrotropin (TSH)	Serum	0.5–5 µIU/mL		0.5–5 µIU/L
triiodothyronine (T_3)		80–200 ng/dL	0.0154	1.23–3 of nmol/L

	Specimen	Conventional	Factor	SI Units
Transferases				
aspartate aminotransferase (AST or SGOT)	Serum	8–33 U/L at 37°C	1	8–33 U/L at 37°C
alanine aminotransferase (ALT or SGPT)	Serum	4–36 U/L at 37°C	1	4–36 U/L at 37°C
gamma-glutamyl-transferase (GGT)	Serum	5–40 IU/L at 37°C	1	5–40 U/L at 37°C
Triglycerides (see Chap. 12)	Serum	10–190 mg/dL	0.01129**	0.11–2.15 mmol/L
Troponin I	Serum	0–0.6 mg/mL		0–0.6 μg/L
Troponin T	Serum	0–0.1 μg/L		0–0.1 μg/L
Urea nitrogen	Serum	8–23 mg/dL	0.357	2.9–8.2 mmol/L
Urea clearance	Serum and urine			
maximum clearance		64–99 mL/min	0.01667	1.07–1.65 L/s
standard clearance		41–65 mL/min, or more than 75% of normal clearance		0.68–1.08 L/s or more than 0.75 of normal clearance
Uric acid	Serum			
male		4.0–8.5 mg/dL	0.05948	0.24–0.51 mmol/L
female		2.7–7.3 mg/dL		0.16–0.43 mmol/L
Vitamin A	Serum	15–60 μg/dL	0.03491	0.52–2.09 μmol/L
Vitamin A tolerance	Serum			
	fasting 3 h or 6 h after 5000 units Vitamin A/kg	15–60 μg/dL	0.03491	0.52–2.09 μmol/L
	24 h	200–600 μg/dL	—	6.98–20.95 μmol/L
		Fasting values or slightly above		Fasting values or slightly above

Table continued on following page

A–1 □ WHOLE BLOOD, SERUM, AND PLASMA CHEMISTRY Continued

Component	System	Typical Reference Intervals		
		Conventional Units	Factor*	Recommended SI Units†
Vitamin B$_{12}$	Serum	160–950 pg/mL	0.7378	118–701 pmol/L
Unsaturated vitamin B$_{12}$–binding capacity	Serum	1000–2000 pg/mL	0.7378	738–1475 pmol/L
Vitamin C	Plasma	0.6–1.6 mg/dL	56.78	34–91 µmol/L
Xylose absorption	Serum			
normal		25–40 mg/dL between 1 and 2 h	0.06661	1.67–2.66 mmol/L between 1 and 2 h
in malabsorption		Maximum approximately 10 mg/dL		Maximum approximately 0.67 mmol/L
		Dose: adult 25 g D-xylose children 0.5 g D-xylose/kg		
Zinc	Serum	50–150 µg/dL	0.1530	7.7–23.0 µmol/L

From Henry JB: Clinical Diagnosis and Management by Laboratory Methods, 19th ed. Philadelphia, WB Saunders Co, 1996, Appendix.

*Factor = number factor (notice that units are not presented).

†Value in SI units = value in conventional units × factor.

‡Usually not measured in blood (preferred specimen is urine, hair, or nails except in acute cases, when gastric contents are used).

§Unit based on hydrogen-ion concentration.

∥As cortisol.

¶As DHEA.

**As triolein.

††One International Unit of insulin corresponds to 0.04167 mg of the fourth International Standard (a mixture of 52% beef insulin and 48% pig insulin).

A–2 □ HEMATOLOGY

Component	Conventional Units	Factor	Recommended SI Units
		Typical Reference Intervals	
Red cell volume			
male	20–36 mL/kg body weight	0.001	0.020–0.036 L/kg body weight
female	19–32 mL/kg body weight		0.019–0.032 L/kg body weight
Plasma volume			
male	25–43 mL/kg body weight	0.001	0.025–0.043 L/kg body weight
female	28–45 mL/kg body weight		0.028–0.045 L/kg body weight
Coagulation and hemostatic tests			
bleeding time	Depends on location and orientation of cut and on particular device, typically 2–8 min		
Activated partial thromboplastin time (APTT)	Depends on activator and phospholipid reagents used, typically 25–35 s		
Antithrombin III			
immunologic	20–30 mg/dL	10	200–300 mg/L
functional	80–120 U/dL	10	800–1200 U/L

Table continued on following page

A–2 □ HEMATOLOGY *Continued*

Component	Conventional Units	Typical Reference Intervals Factor	Recommended SI Units
Clot lysis time			
euglobulin factor	1½–4 h at 37°C		
whole blood	None by 24 h at 37°C		
Clot retraction	Complete by 4 h at 37°C		
Coagulation factors	0.50–1.50 U/mL	1000	500–1500 U/L
Factor XIII (screening test)	Clot insoluble in 5 mol/L urea at 24 h		
Fibrinogen	200–400 mg/dL	0.01	2.0–4.0 g/L
Fibrin(ogen) degradation products			
serum FDP	<10 μg/ml	1	<10 mg/L
plasma D-dimers	<200 ng/mL	1	<200 μg/L
Plasminogen			
immunologic	10–20 mg/dL	10	100–200 mg/L
functional	80–120 U/dL	10	800–1200 U/L
Protein C	70–140 U/dL	10	700–1400 U/L
Protein S (total)	70–140 U/dL	10	700–1400 U/L
Prothrombin time	Depends on thromboplastin reagent used, typically 10–13 s		
Thrombin time	Depends on concentration of thrombin reagent used, typically 17–25 s		

von Willebrand factor		
immunologic	50–150 U/dL	10	500–1500 U/L
ristocetin cofactor activity	50–150 U/dL	10	500–1500 U/L
Complete blood count (CBC)		
hematocrit		
male	41.5–50.4%	0.01	Volume fraction: 0.415–0.504
female	35.9–44.6%		0.359–0.446
hemoglobin		
male	14.0–17.5 g/dL	10	140–175 g/L
female	12.3–15.3 g/dL		123–153 g/L
red cell count		
male	$4.5–5.9 \times 10^6/\mu L$	10^6	$4.5–5.9 \times 10^{12}/L$
female	$4.5–5.1 \times 10^6/\mu L$	10^6	$4.1–5.1 \times 10^{12}/L$
white cell count	$4.4–11.0 \times 10^3/\mu L$	10^6	$4.4–11.3 \times 10^9/L$
Erythrocyte indices		
mean corpuscular volume (MCV)	$80–96 \ \mu m^3$	1	80–96 fL
mean corpuscular hemoglobin (MCH)	27.5–33.2 pg	1	27.5–33.2 pg
Mean corpuscular hemoglobin concentration (MCHC)	33.4–35.5%	0.01	Concentration fraction: 0.334–0.355

Table continued on following page

A–2 □ HEMATOLOGY *Continued*

Component	*Conventional Units*		*Factor*	*Recommended SI Units*	
	Mean percent	**Range of absolute counts**		**Mean number fraction***	**Range of absolute count**
White blood cell differential (adult)					
segmented neutrophils	56%	1800–7800/μL	10^6	0.56	$1.8–7.8 \times 10^9$/L
bands	3%	0–700/μL	10^6	0.03	$0–0.70 \times 10^9$/L
eosinophils	2.7%	0–450/μL	10^6	0.027	$0–0.45 \times 10^9$/L
basophils	0.3%	0–200/μL	10^6	0.003	$0–0.20 \times 10^9$/L
lymphocytes	34%	1000–4800/μL	10^6	0.34	$1.0–4.8 \times 10^9$/L
monocytes	4%	0–800/μL	10^6	0.04	$0–0.80 \times 10^9$/L
Hemoglobin A_2	1.5–3.5% of total hemoglobin		0.01	mass fraction: 0.015–0.035 of total hemoglobin	
Hemoglobin F	<2%		0.01	mass fraction: <0.02	

Typical Reference Intervals

Osmotic fragility

	% Lysis		% NaCl—171 % Lysis—0.01	% Lysed Fraction		
NaCl % (w/v)	Fresh	24 h at 37°C		NaCl mmol/L	Fresh	24 h at 37°C
0.2	—	95–100		34.2	—	0.95–1.00
0.3	97–100	85–100		51.3	0.97–1.00	0.85–1.00
0.35	90–99	75–100		59.8	0.90–0.99	0.75–1.00
0.4	50–95	65–100		68.4	0.50–0.95	0.65–1.00
0.45	5–45	55–95		77.0	0.05–0.45	0.55–0.95
0.5	0–6	40–85		85.5	0–0.06	0.40–0.85
0.55	—	15–70		94.1	0	0.15–0.70
0.6	—	0–40		102.6	—	0–0.40
0.65	—	0–10		111.2	—	0–0.10
0.7	—	0–5		119.7	—	0–0.05
0.75	—	0		128.3	—	0

Platelet count	150,000–450,000/µL		10^6	150–450 × 10^9/L	
Reticulocyte count	0.5–1.5%		0.01	number fraction: 0.005–0.015	
	25,000–75,000 cells/µL		10^6	25–75 × 10^9/L	

Table continued on following page

A–2 □ **HEMATOLOGY** *Continued*

Component	Typical Reference Intervals		
	Conventional Units	*Factor*	*Recommended SI Units*
Sedimentation rate (ESR) (Westergren)			
men under 50 years	<15 mm/h		
men 50–85 years	<20 mm/h		
men over 85 years	<30 mm/h		
women under 50 years	<20 mm/h		
women 50–85 years	<30 mm/h		
women over 85 years	<42 mm/h		
Viscosity	1.4–1.8 times water	1	1.4–1.8 times water
Zeta sedimentation ratio	41–54%	0.01	fraction: 0.41–0.54

From Henry JB: Clinical Diagnosis and Management by Laboratory Methods, 19th ed. Philadelphia, WB Saunders Co, 1996, Appendix.
*All percentages are multiplied by 0.01 to give fraction.

A–3 □ URINE

		Typical Reference Intervals		
Component	Type of Urine System	Conventional Units	Factor*	Recommended SI Units†
Acetoacetic acid	Random	Negative	—	Negative
Acetone	Random	Negative	—	Negative
Addis count	12 h collection	WBC and epithelial cells: 1,800,000/12 h	1	1.8×10^6/12 h
		RBC 500,000/12 h	1	0.5×10^6/12 h
		Hyaline casts: <5000/12 h	1	$<5.0 \times 10^3$/12 h
Albumin				
qualitative	Random	Negative	—	Negative
quantitative	24 h	15–150 mg/d	0.001	0.015–0.150 g/d
Aldosterone	24 h	2–26 μg/d	2.774	6–72 nmol/d
Alkaptone bodies	Random	Negative	—	Negative
α-Amino acid nitrogen	24 h	100–290 mg/d	0.07139	7.1–20.7 mmol/d
δ-Aminolevulinic acid	Random			
	adult	0.1–0.6 mg/dL	76.26	8–46 μmol/L
	children	<0.5 mg/dL		<38 μmol/L
Ammonia nitrogen	24 h	1.5–7.5 mg/d	7.626	11–57 μmol/d
	24 h	20–70 mEq/d	1	20–70 mmol/d
		500–1200 mg/d	0.07139	35.6–85.7 mmol/d
Amylase	2 h	35–260 Somogyi units/h	0.1850	6.5–48.1 U/h

See footnotes on p. 299.

Table continued on following page

A–3 □ **URINE** Continued

Component	Type of Urine System	Conventional Units	Factor*	Recommended SI Units†
				Typical Reference Intervals
Arsenic	24 h	<50 μg/L	0.01335	<0.67 μmol/L
Ascorbic acid	Random	1–7 mg/dL	56.78	57–397 μmol/L
	24 h	>50 mg/d	5.678	>284 μmol/d
Bence Jones protein	Random	Negative	—	Negative
Beryllium	24 h	<0.05 μg/d	111.0	<5.55 nmol/d
Bilirubin, qualitative	Random	Negative	—	Negative
Blood, occult	Random	Negative	—	Negative
Borate	24 h	<2 mg/L	16.44	<32 μmol/L
Calcium				
qualitative (Sulkowitch)	Random	1+ turbidity	1	1+ turbidity
quantitative	24 h			
	average diet	100–240 mg/d	0.02495	2.5–6.0 mmol/d
	low-calcium diet	<150 mg/d		<3.7 mmol/d
	high-calcium diet	240–300 mg/d		6.0–7.5 mmol/d
Catecholamines	Random	<14 μg/dL	59.11*	<828 nmol/L
	24 h	<100 μg/d (varies with activity)	5.911*	<591 nmol/d
epinephrine		<10 ng/d	5.458	<55 nmol/d
norepinephrine		<100 ng/d	5.911	<591 nmol/d
total free catecholamines		4–126 μg/d	5.911*	24–745 nmol/d
total metanephrines		0.1–1.6 mg/d	5.458†	0.5–8.7 μmol/d

Test	Condition	Conventional	Factor	SI
Chloride	24 h	140–250 mEq/d	1	140–250 nmol/d
Concentration test (Fishberg)	Random—after fluid restriction			
specific gravity		>1.025	1	>1.025
osmolality		>850 mOsm/kg	1	>850 mmol/kg
Copper	24 h	<50 μg/d	0.01574	<0.8 μmol/d
Coproporphyrin	Random			
adult		3–20 μg/dL	15.27	46–305 nmol/L
	24 h			
adult		50–160 μg/d	1.527	76–244 nmol/d
child		<80 μg/d		<122 nmol/d
Creatine	24 h			
male		<40 mg/d	7.625	<305 μmol/d
female		<100 mg/d		<763 μmol/d
		Higher in children and during pregnancy	—	Higher in children and during pregnancy
Creatinine	24 h			
male		20–26 mg/kg/d	8.840	177–230 μmol/kg/d
		1.0–2.0 g/d	8.840	8.8–17.7 mmol/d
female		14–22 mg/kg/d	8.840	124–195 μmol/kg/d
		0.8–1.8 g/d	8.840	7.1–15.9 mmol/d
Cystine, qualitative	Random	Negative		Negative
Cystine and cysteine	24 h	10–100 mg/d	4.161‡	42–416 μmol/d
Dehydroepiandrosterone	24 h			
male		0.2–2.0 mg/d	3.467	0.7–6.9 μmol/d
female		0.2–1.8 mg/d		0.7–6.2 μmol/d
Diacetic acid	Random	Negative	—	Negative
Epinephrine	24 h	<20 μg/d	5.458	<109 nmol/d

Table continued on following page

A–3 □ URINE Continued

Component	Type of Urine System	Conventional Units	Typical Reference Intervals		
			Factor*	Recommended SI Units†	
Estrogens total	24 h				
	male	5–18 µg/d	3.468§	17–62 nmol/d	
	female				
	ovulation	28–100 µg/d		97–347 nmol/d	
	luteal peak	22–80 µg/d		76–364 nmol/d	
	at menses	4–25 µg/d		14–87 nmol/d	
	pregnancy	Up to 45,000 µg/d	0.003468	Up to 156 µmol/d	
	postmenopausal	Up to 10 µg/d	3.468	Up to 35 nmol/d	
fractionated	24 h, nonpregnant, midcycle				
estrone (E₁)	—	2–25 µg/d	3.699	7–93 nmol/d	
estradiol (E₂)	—	<10 µg/d	3.671	<37 nmol/d	
estriol (E₃)	—	2–30 µg/d	3.468	7–104 nmol/d	
Fat, qualitative	Random	Negative	—	Negative	
FIGLU (N-formiminoglutamic acid)	24 h	<3 mg/d	5.740	<17.2 µmol/d	
Fluoride	after 15 g of L-histidine	4 mg/8 h	52.63	23.0 µmol/8 h	
	24 h	<1 mg/d		<53 µmol/d	

		Conventional	Factor	SI
Follicle-stimulating hormone (FSH)	24 h			
adult		4–25 U/L	1	4–25 IU/L
prepubertal		4–30 U/L	1	4–30 IU/L
postmenopausal		40–50 U/L	1	40–50 IU/L
midcycle		2 × baseline	1	2 × baseline
Fructose	24 h	30–65 mg/d	0.005551	0.17–0.36 mmol/d
Glucose				
qualitative	Random	Negative	—	Negative
quantitative	24 h	0.5–1.5 g/d	1	0.5–1.5 g/d
copper-reducing substances				
total sugars		Average 250 mg/d	1	Average 250 mg/d
glucose		Average 130 mg/d	0.005551	Average 0.72 mmol/d
Gonadotropins, pituitary (FSH and LH)	24 h	10–50 U/L	1	10–50 IU/L
Etiocholanolone	24 h			
male		1.4–5.0 mg/d	3.443	4.8–17.2 µmol/d
female		0.8–4.0 mg/d		2.8–13.8 µmol/d
11-Hydroxyandrosterone	24 h			
male		0.1–0.8 mg/d	3.263	0.3–2.6 µmol/d
female		<0.5 mg/d		<1.6 µmol/d
11-Hydroxyetiocholanolone	24 h			
male		0.2–0.6 mg/d	3.26	0.7–2.0 µmol/d
female		0.1–1.1 mg/d		0.3–3.63 µmol/d
11-Ketoandrosterone	24 h			
male		0.2–1.0 mg/d	3.274	0.7–3.3 µmol/d
female		0.2–0.8 mg/d		0.7–2.6 µmol/d

Table continued on following page

A–3 □ URINE Continued

Component	Type of Urine System	Conventional Units	Factor*	Recommended SI Units†
11-Ketoetiocholanolone	24 h			
	male	0.2–1.0 mg/d	3.274	0.7–3.3 μmol/d
	female	0.2–0.8 mg/d		0.7–2.6 μmol/d
Lactose	24 h	14–40 mg/d	2.291	41–117 μmol/d
Lead	24 h	<100 μg/d	0.004826	<0.48 μmol/d
Magnesium	24 h	6.0–8.5 mEq/d	0.5000	3.0–4.3 mmol/d
Melanin, qualitative	Random	Negative	—	Negative
Mucin	24 h	100–150 mg/d	1	100–150 mg/d
Muramidase (lysozyme)	24 h	1.3–36 mg/d	1	1.3–36 mg/d
Myoglobin				
qualitative	Random	Negative	—	Negative
quantitative	24 h	<4 mg/L	1	<4 mg/L
Osmolality	Random	500–800 mOsm/kg water	1	500–800 mmol/kg
Pentoses	24 h	2–5 mg/kg/d	1	2–5 mg/kg/d
pH	Random	4.6–8.0	1	4.6–8.0
Phenosulfonphthalein (PSP)	Urine timed after 6 mg of PSP IV			Fraction dye excreted:
	15 min	20–50% dye excreted	0.01	0.20–0.50
	30 min	16–24% dye excreted		0.16–0.24
	60 min	9–17% dye excreted		0.09–0.17
	120 min	3–10% dye excreted		0.03–0.10

Phenylpyruvic acid, qualitative	Random	Negative	—	Negative
Phosphorus	Random	0.9–1.3 g/d	32.29	29–42 mmol/d
Porphobilinogen qualitative	Random	Negative	—	Negative
Porphobilinogen quantitative	24 h	<1.0 mg/d	4.420	<4.4 µmol/d
Potassium	24 h	40–80 mEq/d	1	40–80 mmol/d
Pregnancy tests	Concentrated morning specimen	Positive in normal pregnancies or with tumors producing chorionic gonadotropin	—	Positive in normal pregnancies or with tumors producing chorionic gonadotropin
Pregnanediol	24 h			
male		<1.5 mg/d	3.120	<4.7 µmol/d
female				
peak		1–8 mg/d		3–25 µmol/d
pregnancy		1 week after ovulation		1 week after ovulation
child		<50 mg/d	3.120	<156 µmol/d
Pregnanetriol	24 h	Negative	—	Negative
male		0.4–2.4 mg/d	2.972	1.2–7.1 µmol/d
female		0.5–2.0 mg/d		1.5–5.9 µmol/d
child		Up to 1 mg/d		Up to 3 µmol/d
Protein, qualitative	Random	Negative	—	Negative
Reducing substances, total	24 h	40–150 mg/d	1	40–150 mg/d
	24 h	0.5–1.5 mg/d	1	0.5–1.5 mg/d
Sodium	24 h	75–200 mEq/d	1	75–200 mmol/d
Solids, total	24 h	55–70 g/d	1	55–70 g/d
		Decreases with age to 30 g/d	—	Decreases with age to 30 g/d

Table continued on following page

A-3 □ **URINE** *Continued*

| | | Typical Reference Intervals | | |
Component	Type of Urine System	Conventional Units	Factor*	Recommended SI Units†
Specific gravity	Random	1.016–1.022 (normal fluid intake)	1	Relative density (U 20°C/water 20°C) 1.016–1.022 (normal fluid intake)
		1.001–1.035 (range)		1.001–1.035 (range)
Sugars (excluding glucose)	Random	Negative	—	Negative
Titratable acidity	24 h	20–50 mEq/d	1	20–50 mmol/d
Urea nitrogen	24 h	6–17 g/d	35.70	214–607 mmol/d
Uric acid	24 h	250–750 mg/d	0.005948	1.5–4.5 mmol/d
Urobilinogen	2 h	0.3–1.0 Ehrlich units	1	0.3–1.0 U
	24 h	0.05–2.5 mg/d or	1.693	0.1–4.2 μmol/d
		0.5–4.0 Ehrlich units/d	1	0.5–4.0 U/d

Uropepsin	Random 24 h	15–45 units/h (Anson) 1500–5000 units/d (Anson)	7.37	111–332 U/h 11–37 kU/h
Uroporphyrins				
qualitative	Random	Negative	—	Negative
quantitative	24 h	10–30 μg/d	1.204	12–36 nmol/d
Vanillylmandelic acid (VMA)	24 h	1.5–7.5 mg/d	5.046	7.6–37.9 μmol/d
Volume, total	24 h	600–1600 mL/d	0.001	0.6–1.6 L/d
Zinc	24 h	0.15–1.2 mg/d	15.30	2.3–18.4 μmol/d

From Henry JB: Clinical Diagnosis and Management by Laboratory Methods, 19th ed. Philadelphia, WB Saunders Co, 1996, Appendix.
*As norepinephrine.
†As normetanephrine.
‡Based on cystine.
§Based on estriol.

A–4 □ CEREBROSPINAL FLUID

Typical Reference Intervals

Component	Conventional Units	Factor	Recommended SI Units
Albumin	<10–30 mg/dL	10	100–300 mg/L
Cell count	<5 cells μL	10^6	<5 × 10^6/L
Glucose	40–80 mg/dL	0.05551	2.8–4.4 mmol/L
Lactate dehydrogenase (LD)	Approximately 10% of serum level	—	Activity fraction: approximately 0.1 of serum level
Proteins	12–60 mg/dL	10	120–600 mg/L
Protein electrophoresis			
prealbumin	2–7%	0.01	Fraction: 0.2–0.07
albumin	56–76%		0.56–0.76
alpha-1 globulin	2–7%		0.02–0.07
alpha-2 globulin	4–12%		0.04–0.12
beta globulin	8–18%		0.08–0.18
gamma globulin	3–12%		0.03–0.12
Xanthochromia	Negative	—	Negative

From Henry JB: Clinical Diagnosis and Management by Laboratory Methods, 19th ed. Philadelphia, WB Saunders Co, 1996, Appendix.

A–5 □ AMNIOTIC FLUID

Typical Reference Intervals

Component	Conventional Units	Factor	Recommended SI Units
Appearance			
early gestation	Clear	—	Clear
term	Clear or slightly opalescent	—	Clear or slightly opalescent
Albumin			
early gestation	0.39 g/dL	10	3.9 g/L
term	0.19 g/dL		1.9 g/L
Bilirubin			
early gestation	<0.075 mg/dL	17.10	<1.3 μmol/L
term	<0.025 mg/dL		<0.41 μmol/L
Chloride			
early gestation	Approximately equal to serum chloride	—	
term	Generally 1–3 mEq/L lower than serum chloride	1	Generally 1–3 mmol/L lower than serum chloride
Creatinine			
early gestation	0.8–1.1 mg/dL	88.40	71–97 μmol/L
term	1.8–4.0 mg/dL (generally >2 mg/dL)		159–354 μmol/L (generally >177 μmol/L)
Estriol			
early gestation	<10 μg/dL	3.468	<347 nmol/L
term	<60 μg/dL		>2081 nmol/L

Table continued on following page

A–5 □ AMNIOTIC FLUID Continued

Component	Conventional Units	Typical Reference Intervals	
		Factor	Recommended SI Units
Lecithin/sphingomyelin			
early (immature)	<1:1	1	<1:1
term (mature)	>2:1	1	>2:1
Osmolality			
early gestation	Approximately equal to serum osmolality	1	Approximately equal to serum osmolality
term	230–270 mOsm/kg	1	230–270 mmol/kg
P_{CO_2}			
early gestation	33–55 mm Hg	0.1333	4.4–7.3 kPa
term	42–55 mm Hg (increases toward term)		5.6–7.3 kPa (increases toward term)
pH			
early gestation	7.12–7.38	1	7.12–7.38
term	6.91–7.43 (decreases toward term)		6.91–7.43
Protein, total			
early gestation	0.60 ± 0.24 g/dL	10	60 ± 2.4 g/L
term	0.26 ± 0.19 g/dL		2.6 ± 1.9 g/L

Sodium			
early gestation	Approximately equal to serum sodium	1	
term	7–10 mEq/L lower than serum sodium		7–10 mmol/L lower than serum sodium
Staining, cytologic			
Oil Red O			
early gestation	<10%	0.01	Stained fraction: <0.1
term	>50%		>0.5
Nile Blue Sulfate			
early gestation	0	0.01	Stained fraction: <0.0
term	>20%		>0.2
Urea			
early gestation	18.0 ± 5.9 mg/dL	0.1665	3.00 ± 0.98 mmol/L
term	30.3 ± 11.4 mg/dL		5.04 ± 1.90 mmol/L
Uric acid			
early gestation	3.72 ± 0.96 mg/dL	59.48	221 ± 57 μmol/L
term	9.90 ± 2.23 mg/dL		589 ± 133 μmol/L
Volume			
early gestation	450–1200 mL	0.001	0.45–1.2 L
term	500–1400 mL (increases toward term)		0.5–1.4 L (increases toward term)

From Henry JB: Clinical Diagnosis and Management by Laboratory Methods, 19th ed. Philadelphia, WB Saunders Co, 1996, Appendix.

A–6 □ SYNOVIAL FLUID

	Typical Reference Intervals		
Component	*Conventional Units*	*Factor*	*Recommended SI Units*
Blood-serum-synovial fluid glucose difference	<10 mg/dL	0.05551	<0.56 mmol/L
Differential cell count	Granulocytes <25% of nucleated cells	0.01	Granulocyte number fraction: <0.25 of nucleated cells
Fibrin clot	Absent	—	Absent
Mucin clot	Abundant	—	Abundant
Nucleated cell count	<200 cells/μL	10^6	<200 × 10^6 cells/L
Viscosity	High	—	High
Volume	<3.5 mL	0.001	<0.0035 L

From Henry JB: Clinical Diagnosis and Management by Laboratory Methods, 19th ed. Philadelphia, WB Saunders Co, 1996, Appendix.

A–7 □ GASTRIC FLUID

	Typical Reference Intervals		
Component	*Conventional Units*	*Factor*	*Recommended SI Units*
Fasting residual volume	20–100 mL	0.001	0.02–0.10 L
pH	<2.0	1	<2.0
Basal acid output (BAO)*	0–6 mEq/h	1	0–6 mmol/h
Maximum acid output (MAO) (after histamine stimulation)	5–40 mEq/h	1	5–40 mmol/h
BAO/MAO ratio	<0.4	1	<0.4

From Henry JB: Clinical Diagnosis and Management by Laboratory Methods, 19th ed. Philadelphia, WB Saunders Co, 1996, Appendix.
*Varies between male and female and ages.

A–8 □ MISCELLANEOUS

		Typical Reference Intervals		
Component	Specimen	Conventional Units	Factor	Recommended SI Units
Bile, qualitative	Random stool	Negative in adults	—	Negative in adults
		Positive in children	—	Positive in children
Chloride	Sweat	4–60 mEq/L	1	4–60 mmol/L
Clearances	Serum and urine (timed)			
creatinine, endogenous		115 ± 20 mL/min	0.01667	1.92 ± 0.33 mL/s
Diodrast		600–720 mL/min		10.00–12.00 mL/s
inulin		100–150 mL/min		1.67–2.50 mL/s
PAH		600–750 mL/min		10.00–12.50 mL/s
Diagnex Blue (tubeless gastric analysis)	Urine	Free acid present	—	Free acid present
Fat	Stool, 72 h			
total fat		<5 g/24 h	1	<5 g/d
		10–25% of dry matter	0.01	Mass fraction:
				0.1–0.25 of dry matter
neutral fat		1–5% of dry matter	0.01	0.01–0.05 of dry matter
free fatty acids		5–13% of dry matter	0.01	0.05–0.13 of dry matter
combined fatty acids		5–15% of dry matter	0.01	0.05–0.15 of dry matter
Nitrogen, total	Stool, 24 h	10% of intake	0.01	Mass fraction: 0.1 of intake
		1–2 g/24 h	71.39	71–143 mmol/d
Sodium	Sweat	10–80 mEq/L	1	10–80 mmol/L
Trypsin activity	Random, fresh stool	Positive (2+ to 4+)	—	Positive (2+ to 4+)
Thyroid ^{131}I uptake		7.5–25% in 6 h	0.01	fraction uptake: 0.075–0.25 in 6 h
Urobilinogen				
qualitative	Random stool	Positive	—	Positive
quantitative	Stool, 24 h	40–200 mg/24 h	1.693	68–339 μmol/d
		80–280 Ehrlich units/24 h		

From Henry JB: Clinical Diagnosis and Management by Laboratory Methods, 19th ed. Philadelphia, WB Saunders Co, 1996, Appendix.

B □ COMMON FIXATIVES IN SURGICAL PATHOLOGY

Fixative	Comments
B5	Mercury based; enhances nuclear morphology; tissues become brittle on prolonged exposure (should not exceed 4 hours); leaves mercury pigment (brown) on slides unless treated with iodine and sodium thiosulfate
Bouin's	Contains picric acid and glacial acetic acid; used for soft delicate tissues, e.g., testicular biopsy specimens, GI biopsy specimens; stains tissues yellow; prevents marking ink from washing away (acetic acid does the same)
Ethanol	70% ethanol may be used to dissolve lipids and is suitable for fixing fatty specimens
Formalin	General fixative for tissues intended for paraffin embedding; penetrates tissue at ~1 cm per hour; for optimal fixation the volume of formalin should be 10 times the volume of tissue; may be used for electron microscopy, but better fixatives are available
Glutaraldehyde	Fixative for electron microscopy; tissue pieces must be small (1 mm^3) for optimal fixation
Michel's	Fixative for tissues intended for immunofluorescence
Zamboni's	Fixative for light and electron microscopy; may be used for kidney biopsy specimens
Z-Fix	Zinc based; enhances nuclear morphology similar to B5

C □ COMMON EPONYMOUS TESTS AND DETERMINATIONS

Allen test	Test for glucose in urine using Fehling's reagent
	Test for occlusion of radial or ulnar artery (clinical)
Ames test	Test for quantitating mutagenic capacity of potential carcinogens using histidine-dependent *Salmonella* bacteria
Apt test	Nitroprusside strip test for acetoacetic acid
	Alkali denaturation test for detection of fetal hemoglobin in stool or vomitus of infants
Baermann test	Method for recovering nematode larvae (particularly *Strongyloides*) from stool
Beckman assay	Method for measuring amylase using maltotetrose as substrate
Benedict test	Qualitative screening test based on copper reduction for glucose and other sugars in urine
Bethesda assay	Test for detecting inhibitors against specific coagulation factors
Blondheim test	Qualitative test for myoglobin in urine
Bonsignore test	Test for measuring aminolevulinic acid dehydratase for lead intoxication
Bozicevich test	Serologic test for detecting trichinosis
Brand-Legal test	Cyanide-nitroprusside test for cystine in urine
Cambridge Biotech test	Western blot test for HIV
Cartwright test	Staining procedure for detecting hemosiderin in urine
Castañeda technique	Blood culture using a biphasic bottle containing soybean-casein digest medium for isolation of *Brucella*
Chido test	Serologic test for typing C4 component of complement (C4B-Chido); see also Rodgers test
Clark-Collip test	Test for measuring total serum calcium
Clauss assay	Functional assay for fibrinogen
Coombs' test	Antiglobulin test
Dalmau technique	To demonstrate yeast chlamydospores on cornmeal agar
Davidsohn test	See Paul-Bunnell-Davidsohn test
DeRitis ratio	Ratio of aspartate aminotransferase (AST) to alanine aminotransferase (ALT)
Donath-Landsteiner test	Test for paroxysmal cold hemoglobinuria (PCH) wherein complement-dependent antibodies bind to red blood cells at low temperature and cause hemolysis at $37°C$
Ehrlich test	Benzaldehyde test for urobilinogen in urine

Table continued on following page

C □ COMMON EPONYMOUS TESTS
AND DETERMINATIONS *Continued*

Fishberg test	Urine concentration test for renal function
Fouchet test	Test for bilirubin in blood
Francis test	Test for bile acids in urine
Gerhardt test	Ferric chloride test for acetoacetic acid in urine
Gibson-Cooke test	Sweat chloride test for cystic fibrosis
Guthrie test	Screening test for phenylketonuria using a microbiologic assay
Ham test	Acidified serum test for paroxysmal nocturnal hemoglobinuria (PNH)
Hoesch test	Qualitative test for porphobilinogen in urine
Jaffe test	Test for measuring creatinine
Kjeldahl technique	Technique for quantitation of purified proteins by determining the nitrogen content
Kleihauer-Betke test	Acid elution slide test for detection of hemoglobin F
Knott test	Test for microfilariae in blood by lysis of blood, centrifugation, and examination of the stained sediment
Lancefield precipitation test	Precipitation test used to classify and identify streptococci
Legal test	See Brand-Legal test
Liebermann-Burchard test	Test for cholesterol
Lowry assay	Colorimetric assay for measuring protein concentration
Machado-Guerreiro test	Complement-fixation test for Chagas's disease
Mantoux test	Tuberculin skin test (clinical)
Paigen test	Screening test for galactosemia using a microbiologic assay

C □ COMMON EPONYMOUS TESTS
AND DETERMINATIONS *Continued*

Paul-Bunnell-Davidsohn test	Test for serum heterophil antibodies associated with infectious mononucleosis
Perls iron test	Iron stain (Prussian blue reaction) for iron stores in bone marrow
Rodgers test	Serologic test for typing C4 component of complement (C4A-Rodgers); see also Chido test
Rothera test	Test for acetoacetic acid and acetone in urine
Rous test	Staining procedure for detecting hemosiderin in urine
Rubner test	Test for lactose in urine
Sabin-Feldman dye test	Serologic test for toxoplasmosis
Schilling test	Test for gastrointestinal absorption of cobalamin
Staib test	Growth on caffeic acid agar with production of brown pigment for identification of *Cryptococcus*
Tzanck preparation	Cytologic preparation from the base of a vesicular or bullous lesion (for diagnosis of herpes simplex, varicella, pemphigus, etc.)
van de Kamer test	Test for measuring fecal fat
Van Slyke test	Ninhydrin procedure for measuring total amino acids
Voges-Proskauer test	Test for production of acetylmethylcarbinol from glucose in bacterial cultures (used for differentiating members of Enterobacteriaceae)
Watson-Schwartz test	Screening test for porphobilinogen in urine
Weil-Felix test	Serologic test for rickettsial infections (relatively insensitive and nonspecific)

INDEX

A

ABO group discrepancy, causes of, 80*t*

ABO type-specific unit, emergency blood transfusion and, 77–81

Acanthocyte, causes of, 119*t*

Acetaminophen, bone marrow aspiration and, 147

Acid fast culture, description of, 161*t*

Acid phosphatase, physiologic effects of drugs on, 188*t*

Acid-base balance, electrolytes and, 203–206

Acid-fast bacilli, guidelines for reporting smears for, 173*t*

Acid-fast stain, 172–173

Acidemia
  description of, 203
  metabolic, 206
  respiratory, 209

Acidosis, pH and bicarbonate patterns in, 207*t*

ACP; *see* Acid phosphatase

Acquired immunodeficiency syndrome, blood transfusion as source of, 53

Activated protein C, thrombosis associated with, 141

Acute bilateral pyelonephritis, acute renal failure and, 236*t*

Acute chest syndrome, hemapheresis for treatment of, 100*t*

Acute glomerulonephritis, urinalysis abnormalities associated with, 237*t*

Acute immune hemolytic transfusion reaction, 90–91

Acute nonimmune hemolytic transfusion reaction, 91–92

Acute pyelonephritis, urinalysis abnormalities associated with, 237*t*

Acute renal failure, guidelines for therapeutic plasma exchange for, 106

Acute tubular necrosis
  acute renal failure and, 236*t*
  urinalysis abnormalities associated with, 238*t*

ADH; *see* Antidiuretic hormone

Adrenal failure, hyponatremia caused by, 204*t*

Adrenal function, serum corticosteroid responses and, 220*t*

Adrenal steroids, synthesis and metabolism of, 221*f*

Afibrinogenemia, blood components recommended for, 55*t*

AG; *see* Anion gap

Agitation, magnesium deficiency indicated by, 203

Albumin
  characteristics of, 52*t*
  transfusion of, 63–64

Alcoholism, magnesium deficiency associated with, 203

Aldosterone, concentration of, in plasma, 221

Aldosteronism
  plasma aldosterone concentration and, 222
  primary, diagnosis of, 218

ALG; *see* Antilymphocytic globulin

Alkalemia, hypocalcemia associated with, 202

Alkaline phosphatase, physiologic effects of drugs on, 188*t*

Alkalosis, pH and bicarbonate patterns in, 207*t*

ALL; *see* Leukemia, acute lymphoblastic

Allen test, description of, 307

Allergic interstitial nephritis, acute renal failure and, 236*t*

Allergic reaction, hemapheresis and, 107

Allergic transfusion reaction, 93

Allergy, blood components recommended for, 54*t*

Alloantibody
  identification and report of, 71
  multiple, transfusion and, 83–85
  platelet, posttransfusion purpura diagnosis and, 96

t indicates tables.

311

F

FAB scheme; *see* French-American-British scheme
Face, flushed, contaminated blood product reaction indicated by, 94
Factor deficiency, coagulation disorders and, 131
Factor IX, deficiency of, 139, 140
Factor IX concentrate, characteristics of, 51*t*
Factor V, deficiency of, 140
Factor V Leiden
  specimen handling for, 248*t*
  thrombosis and, 141
Factor VII, assay of, 139
Factor VII concentrate, characteristics of, 51*t*
Factor VIII
  deficiency of, 139, 140
  disorders involving, 137*t*–138*t*
  fresh frozen plasma enriched with, 60
  massive transfusion and, 83
Factor VIII inhibitor, hemapheresis for treatment of, 102*t*
Factor X, deficiency of, 140
Factor XI, deficiency of, 139
Family history, hemostasis disorder diagnosis and, 129
Febrile nonhemolytic transfusion reaction, 92–93
Febrile reaction, blood components recommended for, 54*t*
Fecal specimen, virus detection and, 174
Fever
  acute immune hemolytic transfusion reaction indicated by, 90
  after blood transfusion, 53
  blood transfusion reaction indicated by, 88
  contaminated blood product reaction indicated by, 94
  febrile nonhemolytic transfusion reaction indicated by, 92
  platelet refractoriness associated with, 69
  transfusion-related acute lung injury indicated by, 95
FFP; *see* Plasma, fresh frozen
Fibrinogen
  disorders of, 131
  fresh frozen plasma enriched with, 60
Fibrinogen split products, 131
Fibrosis, esophageal, graft-versus-host disease indicated by, 97

Fine-needle aspiration, cytologic examination and, 257–258
FISH; *see* Fluorescent in situ hybridization
Fishberg test, description of, 308
Fixative, common, in surgical pathology, 306
Flaccidity, magnesium toxicity indicated by, 203
Flow cytometry, lymph node protocol and, 265
Fluid management, clinical pathology panels for, 15*t*
Fluorescent in situ hybridization, specimen handling for, 248*t*
Fluorochrome stain, mycobacterial disease diagnosis and, 172
FNA; *see* Aspiration, fine-needle
FNHTR; *see* Febrile nonhemolytic transfusion reaction
Follicle-stimulating hormone, secretion of, 225
Foreign body culture, description of, 163*t*
Fouchet test, description of, 308
Fragile X syndrome, specimen handling for testing for, 249*t*
Francis test, description of, 308
Free-corticol assay, urinary, 217
Free-thyroxine assay, thyroid function assessment and, 217
French-American-British scheme
  acute myeloid leukemia classified with, 152*t*–153*t*
  leukemia classification with, 150–151
Frozen section, intraoperative consultation and, 256, 257
FSH; *see* Follicle-stimulating hormone
FSP; *see* Fibrinogen split products
Fungemia, blood culture for, 160
Fungus
  blood culture for, 160, 166
  specimen collection for, 166
Fungus culture, description of, 163*t*

G

Gastroenteritis, detection of, 174
Gastrointestinal tract, histologic sections and, in autopsy, 262
Gaucher's disease, erythrocytes affected by, 120
Genital culture, description of, 163*t*
Gentamicin, susceptibility testing with, 180*t*